HOW TO A GROUP PRACTICE

THE DEFINITIVE GUIDE TO SUCCESS IN GROUP PRACTICE DENTISTRY

JARED M. VAN ITTERSUM, D.D.S.
ELIAS J. ACHEY, D.M.D.

TRADEMARKS

Apple®, iPod®, iPhone®, and iTunes® are trademarks of Apple, Inc., registered in the U.S. and other countries. Google Docs™, Google Drive™, and Android™ are trademarks of Google, Inc., registered in the U.S. and other countries. Skype® is a registered trademark of Microsoft Corporation. WebEx™ is a registered trademark of Cisco Systems, Inc. GoToMeeting™ is a registered trademark of Citrix Online, LLC. DocuSign® is a registered trademark of DocuSign, Inc. Dropbox™ is a registered trademark of Dropbox, Inc. Campfire and Basecamp software are registered trademarks of Basecamp. Myers-Briggs® logo is a registered trademark of the MBTI® Trust, Inc., in the United States and other countries. DiSC® is a registered trademark of Everything DiSC, a Wiley Brand (formerly Inscape Publishing, Inc., formerly Carlson Learning Company, formerly Performax Systems International.) Caliper Corp® is a registered trademark. Invisalign® is a registered trademark of Align Technology, Inc. All other trademarks are the property of their respective owners and/or their affiliates in the United States or other countries, and may not be used without written permission. The use of these trademarks within this publication were not authorized by, nor is this publication sponsored by or associated with, the trademark owners. Rutherford Publishing House is not associated with any product or vendor mentioned in this book.

Rutherford Publishing House
PO Box 969
Ramseur, NC 27316
www.RutherfordPublishingHouse.com

Cover design: Navigate Creative Works
Book layout/design: Richard E. Spalding

ISBN-10: 0692725016
ISBN-13: 978-0692725016

LEGAL DISCLAIMER

TABLE OF CONTENTS

ACKNOWLEDGEMENTS

To our wonderful wives, Daisy and Ann Claire, and to all our beautiful children, Ariana, Leilani, Margot, Elias III, and Vida.

The true gift of group practice ownership is the freedom it provides to spend as much time with all of you as possible.

INTRODUCTION

"The next 3 to 5 years are a red-hot market for multiple practice ownership." These were the sentiments a Senior VP of one of the largest dental supply companies in the world shared with us in a private meeting at their headquarters in February, 2016.

WHAT LED UP TO THIS

Several factors have created this market and it is important to understand what has led up to this to understand how it might change again. First, the financial crash of 2008 forced many dentists on the verge of retirement to delay their plans as their 401(k) became a 201(k), and they watched their stock values and savings dwindle. This completely toppled the previous prediction that an influx of baby boomer generation dentists would start retiring ten years ago. Add to that the fact that patients put dental services on the wayside and stopped accepting any dental procedures that were not absolutely necessary, and the collection-production values of offices were taking a hit. Decreased production equalled decreased practice values equalled the wrong time to sell.

Now, the economy has recovered enough that these dentists are able to financially retire and we're seeing an enormous number of practices that should have sold on the market several years ago come into play. Add that to the normal predicted influx of late baby boomer generation dentists selling their offices at this time and it compounds this buyers market.

Second, recent dental school graduates are coming out of school in a far more dire financial situation than in the past. Recent grads have upwards of $300,000 in debt and cannot afford to associate in a private practice that doesn't create absolute financial certainty. Furthermore, at times they cannot get loans from a bank with their existing debt load, so they are funneled into working for larger corporate groups to gain experience and pay down their debt. This is delaying their ability to invest in their own practice by several years, and is only adding to the problem of a surplus of practices for sale.

How does this all relate to the massive opportunity this market provides? Well, there's now enough history and a proven track record across many organizations nationwide that multiple practice ownership not only works but is extremely financially lucrative. The concept is no longer in its infancy in the business cycle and a lot of the risks have been figured out and overcome by the early trailblazers. We're now seeing a large segment of the mid-30's to early 50-year-old dentists that already have stability in their solo practice so they're interested in purchasing an additional satellite office or two. They have a strong desire to start creating a residual income beyond what their individual practice provides. In our own experiment with testing different marketing phrases in marketing pieces, we have seen a much higher percentage response rate in dentists responding to inquiries about learning how to become a multiple practice owner than any other solution we provide. In fact, even outside investment firms see the financial stability and financial opportunity of multiple practice ownership, as they are the newest driving force in purchasing and investing in large DSO's.

What does this mean for you? The banks are lending again. The models exist. The buyers market has been created. Now is the time to become a multiple practice owner.

Jared M. Van Ittersum, D.D.S.
Elias J. Achey, D.M.D.
Founders – Infinity Dental

1

OUR STORY

It was 2008, we were both fresh out of school, had no money whatsoever to work with and were facing the worst recession the nation had seen in 80 years. That's when we started to become multiple practice owners. We've said it a thousand times, "If we can do it, anyone can do it!" We had no experience, no roadmap, no guidance, just trial and error and a vision that was relentless.

It began with creating the perfect partnership. So many people had warned us about getting into a partnership in business and had told us all the horror stories of failed partnerships, but we spent the time to really get our core values and our vision aligned before we signed on the dotted line. And the one thing we can say is we would never have gotten to where we are today without partnership. We have so many memories of dark times, struggles, and fearful situations that we've realized if we didn't have each other as war buddies, as partners, with skin in the game, where each other's success relied on the partnership, I don't think we would have become as successful as we have today.

When you're talking about purchasing multimillion dollar practices and taking on huge responsibilities, that's where skin in the game partnerships really matter. Management companies and consulting service companies have the opportunity to walk away. If you can find somebody whose fate is intertwined with yours, where they truly have skin-in-the-game, where they will always go to bat for you, where they will work late on Saturday nights, and they will do whatever it takes, then connect and move forward with them, because that mentality alone is invaluable. That is what our partnership has provided.

So while we were developing a great partnership in 2008 with our first two practices together, we also recognized that we were fresh out of school and really had no management experience. We saw how critical knowing your numbers, understanding how to manage your team and putting a vision in place for your practice was, but had no idea how to do it. So we started the journey of interviewing many practice management consulting companies and narrowed our search down to someone who today is still a great icon in the industry, Gary Kadi at Next Level Practice. Next Level Practice had a very different approach towards practice management and team management. Rather than just throwing a lot of systems and tools and pearls at the doctor and the team and saying, "Here you go, do it," they really helped reset the context of the office as a whole and the vision for the team members.

We were fortunate to be early pioneers in Next Level's movement of what is now called Complete Health Dentistry. Complete Health Dentistry is a way to organize what we as doctors know as the oral-systemic connection into a model with which the team members can unite behind and educate patients in a way that makes patients appreciate how dentistry fits into their overall health. This model was widely successful for us in 2009 and 2010. It helped explode our first two office's production and collection numbers. For example, our Whitehall, Michigan office in 2008 did $830,000 in collections prior to starting the program. In 2009, it did $1.5 million in collections and in 2010, it did $2.4 million in collections. That was without advertising, without adding new doctors and new team members. It was merely by implementing the Complete Health Model and uniting our team and patients behind the importance of dentistry in their overall health.

Next Level Practice really helped us deliver the philosophy aspect of our early group practice, but we also realized we needed more help in creating infrastructure. Chris Neibauer of Neibauer Dental Care invited us in 2009 to his first seminar, a truly one-of-a-kind seminar, that he planned on hosting before his retirement. Chris Neibauer owned one practice until he was 62 years old and then did 25 startups in five years. Little did we know, he ended up selling his entire group of 26 practices to Heartland Dental several months after our meeting for $62 million.

We were fortunate enough to be the one small private group that was able to pay Chris for his services and reap the benefits. We paid Chris $25,000 cash to sit down with us for an entire weekend with his entire executive team and our executive team, to go over every detail of what it takes to become a group practice owner. Chris and his team gave us everything, and we mean everything: every document, every contract, every idea, what works, what doesn't, from their perspective and their previous five years of owning and managing multiple offices.

But we saw that it was far too much of a micromanagement and fear-based model. It was extremely checklist-and audit system-based, and we received an absolute plethora of modules on scheduling, running the office by checklists, phone scripts, etc. to integrate into our management model. We realized that it did give us the infrastructure we were seeking, it did give us what we were missing to create an expandable turnkey model, and we certainly paid for the rights to use it, but we had to put our own twist on it to find the right balance of systems and culture. So after a lot of trial and error integrating the new systems, we finally felt ready to expand our vision.

We started purchasing practices around our local two offices over the course of the next two years and expanded our local group to six practices very quickly under The Cluster Rule. We integrated our systems and culture through our own motivational summits. These summits gave a place for doctors and team members to collaborate, to have think tank sessions, and break-out sessions in an environment centered around growth and learning. Our summits were also our crash course in public speaking and acted as a training ground in our careers to get used to standing up in front of a crowd for an entire day.

Our model followed what we call The Cluster Rule, where you have the ability to share resources when the offices are very near each other. You can share marketing resources and even do blanket marketing that facilitates multiple office coverage. You can share team members; For example, if a dental assistant is sick and a nearby office has the ability to share in their capacity, the doctor doesn't have the added stress of having a front desk team member assist that day. We were able to master moving around team members based on our culture of helping each other.

We can't tell you how much of a stress-relief it was as a practicing dentist to know that if one of our hygienists or one of our assistants was sick, there was a very reasonable chance one of our other offices would send a supporting team member over to help us and to know they were trained on the exact same systems that our normal team member was. It also showed us how great our systems were and how frustrating it was to work with people who weren't trained in our systems. When we did have to have a sub from an outside source come and help, for example, a substitute dental hygienist, we would get so frustrated when they didn't understand our systems, and the patient flow and the patient experience wasn't seamless like it normally was.

In fact, things were going so well, profitability was so good and the culture of our organization seemed so complete, that we decided to grow outside of our local West Michigan borders. Looking back, we call our first local phase of growth in the West Michigan area Phase One. We began our Phase Two of growth in 2011 and 2012. We put together a transition team consisting of three individuals who had expertise in national mass marketing and sales. We put together a program to market to dentists in several states in which we were getting licensed. But to do that, we had to overcome some major hurdles. First, we had to figure out a way to finance the purchase of additional offices because the banks were starting to close their doors to adding more debt to our existing load. Second, we had to perfect our systems to remotely train and manage offices that are outside of a daily drive. As you can imagine, these are some pretty big barriers.

In further chapters, we'll go into detail about how we overcame this. But through the spirit of being resourceful, we were able to come up with working business solutions to both, and we were able to start marketing to doctors around the country. We had a vision to create something enormous that would have the ability to exert enormous influence on the industry, but on our terms as practicing doctors fighting to preserve the integrity of dentistry. At that time, we were 29 and 32 years-old and figured we had a very, very long career ahead of us. It was the beginning of a 30-40 year journey, so we said let's go for it!

We purchased an additional nine practices in seven states in fewer than two years, including practices in New York, Kentucky, Pennsylvania, Indiana, Ohio, Alabama and Texas. We threw annual information summits for doctors to fly to us to spend an entire day with our team and understand our company. We would fly to their offices to meet the doctors and their teams. We had these offices come to our own summits. We were crushing it and thought we had it all figured out! Boy, were we wrong, and did we ever get our butts kicked quickly thereafter.

Because no one ever told us what to do and what not to do, we realized that we had not calculated the working capital in our model as accurately as we should have and we had not correctly calculated staging out the purchases of the multiple practices in the right timing. We found ourselves in the situation where we had too many offices coming on too quickly, and the infrastructure could not support it. We very quickly got behind on bills and keeping up with managing the accounts receivables and the cash flow situation that are a result of the transition period. This delicate balance ended up becoming our biggest nightmare.

We remember a very specific point when we were $598,000 *behind* on bills. We were both still practicing full time as clinical dentists and because our debt situation had gotten so bad, we were both the lowest paid doctors out of 19 Infinity Dental doctors. We were literally working to pay everyone else's bills and paychecks. There were many times when we were ready to just throw in the towel, when we would say, "Why are we even doing all of this?" or, "Just managing only one practice would be so much easier."

We have a very specific memory of being in a sauna on a weekend just trying to get away, just sweating it out, shaking our heads and just strategizing and asking ourselves what do we do, what do we have to do. Those were very, very dark days for us and it is a warning to those that want to go down this route and don't know what they're doing. When you have that amount of personnel and doctors to manage, debt flowing and cash to manage, things can get over your head very quickly.

It was our biggest failure. But our mentors inspired us and motivated us to redirect, to have the hard conversations that we had to have with our teams and our doctors, to have integrity with ourselves. Our mentors acted as true partners in guiding us in the right direction to make some very tough decisions. And redirect we did.

We were able to make some tough financial decisions, do some dramatic cost-cutting, sell some of our draining practices and put pride to the side. It took about a year to climb out of the hole, but we were able to do it, and through that create safety nets and infrastructure so that we never get back to that place ever again.

We faced the boogieman and we survived, and it has only made us stronger and more knowledgeable. On a side note, it also made our partnership even stronger. It's amazing how when you're in the trenches and things aren't going well and you stick by each other's side, your partner really, truly does become a war buddy.

One of the people whom we have studied intensely over the years and whose many seminars we have attended is Anthony Robbins. Tony Robbins teaches a concept called the CANI Principle, which stands for Constant And Never Ending Innovation. Look, business is only two things: marketing and innovation. When we were in our dark period years ago, one solution was to give up. The other solution was to be resourceful and innovate new ways to become profitable. We recognized that our infrastructure and business model needed some more innovation and we needed to be resourceful in how we got there. So we took a gladiator-style perspective, pulled all-nighters, did whatever it took and put countless hours into resetting our infrastructure. We created eight divisions of management within our organization to help keep a constant eye on every aspect of our organization.

Furthermore, we co-developed a software solution with our great accounting firm to better manage the numbers on a daily/weekly basis. But most importantly, we reset our integrity as leaders and owners of our organization with our doctors and our teams. We sat down with every single doctor and let them know where we were and what was happening when we were in that dark period. We spoke from our hearts' and we asked them for their help or their forgiveness. And a magical thing happened. Every single one of them stepped up and asked how they could help, that they believed in what we stood for, that they believed they were part of something great and did not want to see it go away.

We refocused on our foundation for the next couple of years, put a halt to all growth and gave our doctors, teams, and company the attention they deserved. Through that, however, we grew more than we ever could have by just adding to the number of practices that we owned. Through halting and refocusing, we were able to create Infinity Dental University. Infinity Dental University is unlike anything the dental industry has ever seen. It became our training program for offices, based on our eight years of experience in how to manage a dental practice and dental teams from a practicing dentist perspective.

By refocusing on our foundation, we were able to recognize just how valuable our core group was. We changed our focus from growing, growing, growing and adding more practices, and we realized that you can have it all, including time and financial freedom, from a small group. This led to the concept of developing our Platinum Partners Program. Platinum Partners is our partnership program that allows dentists to have exactly what we have: freedom. Through this unprecedented program, we're giving away all of our resources so that other dentists can purchase and own practices, yet have partners that have done it before. We can share the risk and can relieve the burden of management - which we know is the trickiest part of owning multiple practices.

There is a classic diagram floating around on the Internet defining success as a series of ups and downs with a gradual upward trend on average; it really hit home for us. It was never easy to get to where we are, and some aspects of it may have involved a lot of luck in the beginning, but most of it was a whole lot of blood, sweat and tears and hard work that most people never knew was even happening in the background.

We've created this book and our programs so that doctors don't have to repeat the same mistakes that we made and have the roadmap that we never had. That is our gift back to dentistry, our ultimate gift back to dentistry.

2

BENEFITS OF
GROUP PRACTICE

Three words: Economies of scale. There are some things you just can't do and take advantage of when you have a single practice. Let us explain. First, you have the ability to get economies of scale in group ordering. We have been with Henry Schein for over eight years now and in 2012 we qualified for what's called Henry Schein Special Markets. By being a member of their Special Markets program, we're in the top 200 D.S.O.s (Dental Service Organization) and have benefits that aren't available to their solo practitioner clients. For example, when you see those big discounts when you order in bulk of a product (e.g. buy 15,000 gloves get 7,500 gloves free), we get those percentage discounts at the single item level.

We also get our own catalog that we custom create with our own selection of products that Henry Schein gives a special pricing on, and also negotiates with their sub-vendors. On average, we save 22-25% on clinical and front office supplies versus their solo practice clientele. It can be hard to appreciate the financial impact of this when you're looking at one practice, but when you multiply those financial benefits times five to ten practices, it becomes a pretty significant savings overall to your bottom line, and can literally come close to replacing your clinical income.

Lab expenses are another great example. We have a ten-year relationship with Mac Dental Lab, a substantial lab out of the Midwest, and co-created a program for our doctors that are a part of Infinity Dental Partners to receive an 18% minimum discount across the board of all lab services. Again, at a solo practice level, this is pretty good, but it becomes fantastic when you multiply this times many doctors and many practices.

A third benefit of economies of scale is negotiating PPOs and insurance rates. It is somewhat difficult to approach an insurance company or PPO to ask or negotiate for better reimbursement when you have one practice. But when you have a group, your ability to negotiate greatly improves. We have started these discussions in the last year and have seen favorable return on getting better reimbursement.

As practicing dentists, we know that we are the largest producers in the office and really do make or break the success of the practice. Yes, we know hygienists and the rest of the team are critical to it, but you have your head in the sand if you don't think that placement and manage-ment of associates and doctors is paramount to the success of a group. That's why we have spent so much time mastering our on-boarding and associate management program, and have developed an entire company around attracting great doctors.

What we found in our early years is that it's very difficult to place a full time doctor in a single office unless that office is growing 30% or more every year. If the senior doctor is not willing to drop a day or two on their schedule to bring in an associate, there's almost no way to offer another doctor four to five days and create a full time schedule to meet their needs. What we have found is that having two to three offices within 30 miles is the optimal way to offer an associate a full time schedule. If those offices are in a normal growth curve, you can offer them two days at one practice and two to three days at the other practice, and instantly give them a full time schedule for them to be able to take care of their families and their needs. Again, this is part of The Cluster Rule.

Without a cluster of practices to facilitate associate placement, most solo practitioners lose the opportunity to find great doctors. This problem will never go away as long as solo practitioners want to continue practice and are not willing to retire and walk away. And there's a huge problem with that model, too. There needs to be a trust transfer from senior doctor to associate doctor and very rarely does that transfer work well when the doctor just retires. The current standard is that you will lose 10% of the active patients during an associate transition when a doctor retires, so it's critical to do everything possible to mitigate that damage.

As mentioned earlier, sharing team members is also a critical benefit of group practice, whether it is a hygienist or a dental assistant, because you don't have to shut down the schedule if someone is sick. Team members really like this group practice benefit and the culture that comes along with it because it alleviates stress. Our experience is that they like having team members from other offices in the group who understand the same systems versus a sub from an agency, when one is needed.

Finally, from our perspective, the number one entrepreneurial benefit of group practice is having multiple residual incomes. This is what allowed us to retire at an early age and have total financial and time freedom. We could never have done it with one practice. In fact, we grew our first practice from $830,000 in annual collections to $2.4 million in collections in less than two years and that was still not enough to be able to retire. However, we have a model that shows that with as few as three practices, you are able to replace your income and retire clinically if that is a goal you seek.

Multiple practice ownership is the answer. Our model has shown that with a cluster group of three practices with approximate $1 million collections per office and a 15% or greater EBITDA, you can replace a $250,000 to $400,000 income based off of the profits of those three offices, and it only gets better as the number of offices increase.

3

LEGAL DOCUMENTS AND PURCHASE MODELS

Legal documents and contract law - some pretty boring, mind-numbing stuff to a practicing dentist - but if you're going to become an entrepreneur, you'd better get very, very comfortable with the concept and get to know contract law very well. At the end of the day, it may save you.

In our nine years, in purchasing 15 dental practices, we've invested a combined total of over $120,000 into the development of our contracts. Over those nine years, we've had three separate law firms work on them and continually update/improve them. We've had 17 law firms from other dentists help create workable revisions that worked for the doctors on their end. So our contracts are a very long evolution of many sets of eyes to create an organic document that now is very fair and can solve almost any issue and protect all parties.

So why is contract law so crucial? Well, beyond the boiler plate B.S., there are some things in contracts that only come up when things go bad. If things are going great, money's coming in, and doctors and teams are happy, contract laws don't make any appreciable difference. In our experience though, when things go bad, contracts are the only thing that matter. Let us explain with a story.

We purchased an office in State X from Doctor Y in 2012. This was after courting and developing a wonderful relationship with the doctor for the previous six months as part of our purchase process. Doctor Y was a wonderful man, a leader within his office and a great dentist. We had gone on several trips together around the country, had met his entire family and even met his parents, who were in end-stage illness at their nursing home. We could not have developed a stronger connection or a stronger brotherhood. We truly cared about each other beyond a business relationship, or so we thought at the time. In some of the earlier stages of our contracts, we had a provision for a doctor to break contract with us at the 24-month point without any consequences if we were unable to secure bank financing after a two-year owner-financed arrangement. We'll get into more detail about our owner financing model later on, but for this story just know that our contracts did not protect us and gave that doctor an out.

So we invested tens of thousands of dollars into equipment. We invested 24 months of our lives. We invested all of our management team overhead. We got a replacement associate doctor lined up. We brought in two specialists, etc. etc. etc. At the 24-month mark, we had the option to continue moving forward with the doctor in the existing relationship. Based on all the conversations, we assumed we were going to continue working together, and his 24-month clause that provided an out would never be enabled. We thought we had done our job and provided him massive value, and assumed that that clause would never be a factor if we performed on our end.

We thought the brotherhood we created would trump all, but that little clause that his attorney put in our contracts (that allowed him to walk away at 24 months and retain 100% of his practice and all of his assets) came up in a letter one month prior to the 24-month mark. In this letter he let us know his intent to take his practice back, that he appreciated everything we'd done for him, but he was going to retain it and put it back on the open market. You can only imagine the feeling in our stomachs and in our hearts, and the betrayal that we felt. But the reality is we weren't protected as buyers. The reality is that unfortunately we live in a business world, and you can't rely on your relationships and on your hand shakes as much as in previous generations, as our parents and our grandparents had taught us. We were foolish and naive to think that that clause would not ever come up as an option. When it did, it didn't matter; all the blood, sweat and tears we had spent providing massive value meant nothing. Our relationship didn't matter, the only thing that mattered was contract law. And doctor Y, sure enough, walked away from our organization with all of his assets, all of the investments we put into his office that negated any income to us, and left us in the dust.

So again, when the going gets tough, contract law is all that matters. Learn from our mistakes! Make sure you're protected and do not rely on the relationships to trump what is the written word.

Let's talk about fairness in documents as a critical factor. When we developed our 50-50 program, we had to develop an additional set of documents to supplement it. When our law firm created this new set of documents, they weighed them more towards Infinity Dental Partners in terms of protection, and let us tell you about the storm that created. The two of us created our partnership in 2009 as a true 50-50 deal where everything is split down the middle and everything, even on paper, looks very fair. In the development of our new program, the moment that we started weighing things to favor us more if the going got tough, all hell broke loose with the prospective offices. We actually lost two purchases (read: lost two $1.5 million dollar offices) that we had been communicating with for a very long time and with whom we had developed a very good relationship, all because our 50-50 contracts were too weighted on our end. We can tell you right now that attorneys will always try to sway the power in one direction, but don't do it. 50-50 contracts have to provide absolutely equal protection. It doesn't matter if you're bigger than them in terms of your size and capacity. Things have to be equal or the relationship will not move forward.

So in regard to our 50-50 partnership, what has made it a successful structure is a fantastic operating agreement. Operating agreements in 50-50 partnerships are the most important thing. Here's why: In a partnership, collective decisions must be made that would not come up if you owned 100%. One of the most common things we see, for example, is how you make purchases. How do you agree on what to purchase, how to purchase it, and what amount merits a "discussion of purchases" while maintaining an efficient office? We've set it up so that anything below $500 can be purchased without consulting the partners. If there's a purchase above $500, that requires a consult, and we have a specific form that we use to discuss that piece of technology or equipment briefly and move forward together in unanimous decision.

Finally, let's discuss our associate contracts and what makes them so unique. One of the biggest problems doctors face is keeping an associate on for the long term. It's easy to get an associate excited about an office and support them and onboard them, but the key to a long-term successful group is to keep them happy and successful and growing your office for many years. But how do you do that? You want a motivated associate, but you don't want them so motivated that they want to go off and do their own start-up, or purchase an office from somebody else just outside of their non-compete. That has happened to us several times. To add to the problem, it's very expensive to transition a new associate and takes a long time. The credentialing process alone can take upwards of 8 weeks depending on how many insurance companies your office takes. We have credentialed doctors internally and externally by outsourcing, and the fees can reach as high as $19,000 to credential one associate doctor if you send it out. Obviously, keeping a good, high-producing associate long term is key!

So we created what we call internally our golden handcuffs program (in reality, we call it our associate partnership program). Simply put, it's a profit-sharing plan that creates longevity in our relationship with associates. Our associate profit share plan is a seven-year program. The associate works for the first 24 months based on the 30% collections commission minus 30% of their lab expenses. After 24 months of just a standard contract, we then give the associate 10% of the net operating income in a form of a quarterly bonus check. With this, the associate gets the benefit of ownership and has a performance-based income, but they do not have to purchase any equity; We actually give them that percentage contractually! On year four, they get 15%, on year five they get 20% and on year six, they get 25% of the net operating income. Mind you, they have never had to go to the bank or pull cash out and purchase any of that percentage. It is their gift for their commitment for staying with us. But the numbers work out and it's a small price to pay in terms of what high associate turnover will cost you, which can get very expensive. It's also a motivating factor for them to produce more and keep the overhead low because now they're inherently thinking like an owner. Now they actually care about overhead and want to keep ordering down so that it doesn't affect their percentage of the net operating income.

But that's not all. They can stay indefinitely on the 25% profit share plan and get their quarterly bonus checks; however, they also have the option to purchase at year seven. The equation is designed on a seven-year plan based on purchasing practices on a seven-year note so that the office is free and clear of debt at the time of sale to the associate. The purchase option is also beneficial as it is designed to keep them on the full seven years to help run the office. Furthermore, we evaluate the purchase price at year five, even though the purchase isn't triggered until the end of year seven. The goal is to create positivity equity on day one for the associate, and to create a practice with decreased risk for banks to lend toward. If the office is on a continual increase of collections every year, they will be purchasing an office that has instant equity and is a fantastic value for them at the time of purchase. Banks love it, because they are purchasing an office at a lower cost than what the true value is, and banks like to see that positive equity on day one.

Currently, we've had two associates go to the sixth year since we have implemented this program, and our first doctor is in line to purchase the practice on December 31st, 2016. We can tell you that he's very successful and our associates on this program are major producers. They feel like they have a vision with an end point, and it has truly created a win-win situation with keeping doctors on board and happy for a very long time.

Finally, let's talk about one of our most successful purchase models. What if we told you that you could purchase a practice with no money in the bank and no money down, you could actually completely bypass ever talking to a bank, and the selling doctor would make more money and be happier than with traditional bank financing? In 2009, we created an owner-finance model to purchase practices with zero dollars. There's a unique history to how we created this strategy, and it's applicable to every dentist currently entering the group practice arena. Presently, the most recent statistics we've ascertained are that banks are lending up to about $1.8 million total for private practitioners, which can get you 2 or 3 practices. After that ceiling, it's becoming much harder to get lending unless you are a well-established D.S.O.

We purchased our first five practices in Michigan through traditional bank financing and we did this during the recession when things were already pretty tight. We had maxed out our capacity to get lending with the banks, but in our minds, our growth was only beginning. Bank of America Practice Solutions blatantly told us they were not going to lend anymore and that we couldn't take on any more debt, otherwise they were going to call default on our loans. But you can't tell that to two individuals as hungry as we were with a vision of growing, because when you're not growing, you're dying!

So we contracted with some fantastic dental-specific attorneys and evaluated what plan B would look like to allow us to grow even though the banks had our hands tied. We created a model that contractually allowed us to own the offices, but showed up as zero debt to the banks. We had this evaluated by the banks and got a complete green light for the model! In a nutshell, it's an owner-financing model. Here's how it worked: We evaluated an office on either a seven-year or a ten-year note, and we put it at a high interest rate (which was generally 6.5% to 8% interest). The language of the contracts and the model were such that the first 24 months were treated as a consulting agreement fee, instead of a note-payment fee to the doctor. The purchase price decreased every month by the consulting fee amount, so that at the end of the 24-month period, the purchase price was lowered by 24 payments that came from the cash flow of the office. At that point, the banks agreed that they would be happy to evaluate for a balloon payment, but we also had the additional option to continue owner financing.

Since getting out of that rut in the relationship with the banks, we have continued this model without the consulting agreement format for several offices. An owner-financed model makes so much sense, except for one scenario. If you have a doctor who wants to retire immediately and pull the cash out and use it all at once - perhaps to buy a second home or to pay off debt - the owner-financing model will not work. But if you have a doctor who plans on either being in the office and continuing to work, is young enough where they plan on being around in a normal lifestyle with normal finances for the next seven years, or they don't have anything that needs to be immediately paid off, owner-financing allows the doctor to make so much more money on the office than if a bank financed it. Why do you think banks have such beautiful, large buildings everywhere? It's because they make all of their money off of the interest. If you buy a house over a 30-year mortgage, even at a low fixed interest rate, your total payment is far more than most people realize for the total value of the house. If the doctor has a 7% interest rate on their office on a $750,000 sale, they end up making a staggering amount more during the length of the note versus bank note financing. They'll be taxed by means of ordinary income on the note as it's paid down, but that nearly matches the capital gains that they would be paying to Uncle Sam on a balloon sale.

Here's how the numbers work out: If you have a practice that collected $1 million in the last 12 months and was evaluated at a practice value of $700,000, you would get $700,000 from a bank minus a 10% brokerage fee if you use a broker, netting you $630,000 before taxes. If you owner financed that, you would end up getting $1.15 million before taxes, a $520,000 difference over seven years (as we take no brokerage fee during our acquisitions). Again, that's $520,000 more! Can you imagine what you could do with that additional interest money?

What's exciting about this model is that it eliminates a major step from the equation that generally slows things down: getting banks involved. Anyone who's ever bought a house or received a big loan knows how that can be a pain in the butt and can take a significant amount of time. By circumventing the banks, you can move forward in a business relationship faster and utilize a purchase model where the doctor gets more income than they ever could have traditionally!

4

—

CREATING
INFRASTRUCTURE
AND YOUR
MANAGEMENT TEAM

Buying practices is one thing, managing them is an entirely different can of worms. Anybody can find an office or two to purchase on top of their first practice, but not just anybody can successfully implement a management model that works and is expandable. In this chapter, we're going to talk about creating your own eight divisions of management, and the history of how we created ours. We're also going to show you how to set up a centralized command with bookkeepers and satellite checking systems, and how to set up a centralized AR division to maximize the collections of all of your offices.

We began our management team journey by first hiring a Director of Operations. At the time, our Director of Operations was responsible for running four to five offices, and it worked well enough. But as we grew, we quickly realized we needed more than one person; that the day-to-day tasks were too overwhelming. So we expanded our team to include a Director of Operations and a Senior Facilitator. Our Senior Facilitator was responsible for coaching and teaching of our systems to our teams, while our Director of Operations handled most administrative issues and HR. We then expanded that team of two into an Operations Team of three individuals who were running admin, hiring, and HR. Our Senior Facilitator still continued the coaching and training of our systems into the organization.

Our final model, which we have had for several years now, is by far the most effective and successful. We call it our Eight Divisions of Management. We created Eight Divisions of Management to measure and support every hat that needs to be worn in a successful dental office. We confidently have a set of eyes looking at every aspect from a business standpoint to ensure that culture and solvency thrive within the organization. We created the eight divisions to have accountability and to make sure that we're measuring every aspect that can be measured based on a successful business model. Our Eight Divisions of Management consist of an Executive level, an Administration level, a Marketing level, a Case Acceptance level, a Production level, a Quality Assurance level, a Finances level and a Human Resources level.

Let's take a more detailed look at what the roles and responsibilities of each position are, and you'll see how every single aspect of an office is covered.

EXECUTIVE DIVISION

The Executive division consists of Doctor Elias Achey and Doctor Jared Van Ittersum as the founders of our organization and practicing doctors. We have the primary responsibility of managing the doctors of the practices as CEOs, teaching and coaching how to monitor the vision, culture and solvency of our practices. As CEOs, we must maintain vision, culture and solvency; however, we have learned over the years that culture trumps everything. There are times when a decision may not be the most solvent, and you may have to take a hit for your group, but if it maintains a great culture, sometimes you just have to take one for the team. It's one of the greatest pieces of advice that we can give. Always, always, always make sure that you're providing a world-class culture. Culture trumps solvency and vision. Be rigid with your principals, but flexible with your policies.

We've been amazed at the way the simplest little thing can upset a team member and can spread like wild fire throughout your organization. There are rarely any times where money is more important than culture. When you're running a group in the 21st century, where all team members can easily communicate with each other, mark our words, they will. Gossip, no matter how strict your policies are (and we mandate immediate termination if you gossip!), occurs within a group practice setting just as much if not more than in solo practice.

Additionally, as the Executive division, we provide leadership coaching to doctors based on the lessons that we have learned from coaches and experiences practicing and managing multiple locations. We created a new associate training program that's facilitated by flying the doctors in to our centralized location prior to placement in an office. They interview with Doctor Van Ittersum and Doctor Achey, tour our local West Michigan offices of Infinity Dental Partners, take a Kolbe profile test to test their personality traits and learn the philosophies of Infinity Dental Partners. Having another practicing dentist who is central to on-boarding new associates early on is mandatory.

ADMINISTRATION DIVISON

The Administration division is responsible for having the right people in the right places with the right equipment. When a new team member is hired, or there is a need for a hire for an office, the Administration division directs placement of any advertising for a new employee with the Human Resources division, and administrates and assists the local team leader in a five-step process of hiring. This includes a telephone interview, or WebEx tele-video conference, scheduling an on-site second interview with a team member or with the team leader, administering a Kolbe test and interpreting the results, following up with two book reports we require prior to placement, and final checking and following through with all licensure and Human Resources related processes.

If new team members require additional training, the Administrative division evaluates what specific weak-nesses the team members possess and provides training in the following ways: First, they facilitate onsite peer-to-peer training with an existing team member and we pay those existing team members an increased training wage of an additional $5 per hour. Second, they coordinate online WebEx-based training with team members from other IDP offices. Again, this is a huge benefit of group practice. Third, they coordinate any specialty software equipment processes training with any third party support companies, such as Dentrix. Finally, they coordinate with IDP's Education Facilitator if the training is related to modules within Infinity Dental University. This coordination allows for team members to gain access to our video library of training videos and get caught up quickly per position.

The Administration division in Infinity Dental Partners provides three on-site annual visits to the office for in-person training. We've found over the years that even with the best remote management model, team members and doctors appreciate some love and connection with their support team throughout the year. We keep it to three visits to control overhead and make it manageable.

Administration oversees all equipment audits, new major equipment orders and equipment support related issues. Administration division oversees a master schedule for the practice to coordinate any Infinity Dental Partners related events, to coordinate vacation schedules for the doctors and team members and to assist in the coordination of substitute doctor and team members to continue the normal ebb and flow of the practice. This is absolutely critical to make sure that you have predictable monthly collections for your group. For example, there was a year in our infancy when we didn't control the master calendar as well as we should. Along came the holiday season in December, and most of our offices and most of our doctors took off more than a week. However, bills don't stop coming just because the offices shut down, and they can take a production producing machine quickly to zero! That year the organization lost over $300,000 around the holidays, and we had to do a cash crunch to make sure the bills were paid, all because we didn't plan ahead with a master calendar. We didn't ensure we had substitute doctors and team members to cover the offices, or at the very least, stagger schedules on vacation time between the offices. It's a very bad thing for cash flow when all of the offices close for an extended time all at once. Don't ever let it happen!

QUALITY ASSURANCE DIVISION

Quality Assurance division is there to make sure your patients are being served in a world-class way and your team members are happy. They schedule a monthly one-page anonymous review that is filled out by team members and mailed directly to the the corporate office to get an honest, on-the-ground perspective of the pulse of the practice at all times. To ensure a world-class patient experience, Quality Assurance audits online reviews and makes unscheduled phone screening calls to assess the first point of contact for the office, and see where coaching opportunities are available.

Once per quarter, Quality Assurance facilitates a Flip video-recorded role-playing session in which the teams block a two-hour session to practice the entire patient experience from front to back and out the door. It's mandatory for the doctor to be there to hear the language used and see the physiology present of each team member.

A goal for the office of 95% patient retention is established, and Quality Assurance facilitates a checklist audit system to tell us the number of patients lost and why. A quarterly audit on active patient count against patient retention provides feedback on when we may need marketing to reactivate patients externally. Quality Assurance oversees that the online reviews favor the hygiene experience, and manages an agreement with team leaders to review online reviews one time per day and actively respond to negative reviews online within 24 hours.

MARKETING DIVISION

Marketing division helps analyze the capacity of an office and define the most effective marketing strategies for the demographics of the office. Marketing division implements a new internal patient referral program and sets the office up with referral cards and incentives. They coordinate with Quality Assurance division on the patient experience, the cornerstone of a successful internal referral system.

Marketing division, bi-annually, measures the actual capacity of the practice in terms of monthly and annual collections against the potential capacity for collections. Website development/maintenance and a social media foundation are evaluated and managed through Marketing division and our subcontracted company Navigate. If necessary, Marketing division coordinates and is the point of contact for Navigate to create a new website and social media package.

After analyzing the capacity with the other divisions, Marketing division coordinates any external marketing for the office through our subcontracted marketing company, Three Layer Marketing, for any print media direct mailers or internal brochures. Marketing division manages the implementation of our optional iSmile Program, a local community giveback program to help combat child hunger locally through dental office visits.

FINANCE DIVISION

Finance division puts a set of eyes on all things related to the cash flow of the offices and of our group. When an office becomes a part of Infinity Dental Partners as a 50-50 equity partner or a 100% partner, finance division ensures the finances are lined up to cover payroll, offices overhead, bank notes, and doctor's consulting fees, while having put away enough for bonus payout and rainy days.

The division is responsible for payroll services both for team members and for doctors. Payrolls calculated are either direct deposited or mailed every two weeks with a password protected email, allowing team members to view the spreadsheet of the payroll, overtime bonus, hours, etc. Finance division monitors the solvency of each office every month, makes sure cash flow is maximized, and helps calculate the proper drugs and supplies ordering budget, based on the previous month's collections.

Finance division provides these updated numbers through cash-based P&Ls, and provides optics on all financial aspects in the office, both for the executive division of our organization and for the doctor. We've developed a total of three financial dashboards over the years, and Finance division has always input the proper information, along with our dental CPAs, to give us accurate dashboards to get snapshots of the organization. Finance division ensures that the team pay scale is up-to-date by running a quarterly report on percentage incomes to collection ratios, and also reports where the office ranks nationally on the percentage for that region. This provides information to help evaluate raise potentials and hiring information.

Finance division coordinates with Henry Schein Special Markets to ensure the office fee schedules are up to date, and runs one annual report for the office to make sure the office fees are at a minimum of 60% or above for all procedures compared to offices within a ten-mile radius.

HUMAN RESOURCES DIVISION

Human Resources division is responsible for all things related to the administrative part of hiring team members and for managing difficult team member situations. HR also directs the termination of an employee, and sees that all proper documentation is in place surrounding the reason for termination, with documentation of possible redirects or opportunities to improve, releasing documents and exit interviews.

HR directs the new associate dentist credentialing process, processing all necessary insurance credential information, setting out proper time frames to ensure associates and practices are credentialed in a timely manner to ensure proper reimbursement. This aspect of the division is critical! We had an office in Ohio in which we needed to onboard an associate very quickly in order to make the deal work out. Because all of our ducks weren't in a row with credentialing, we lost almost $30,000 in the first month from lost insurance reimbursements!

One final note about HR division. It may seem like they have very few tasks when compared to the overall Eight Divisions of Management, but this division requires a special amount of attention. When we bought our 5th practice and had only a Director of Operations, we ran into a rather unpleasant HR scenario. Almost a year into owning the practice, we had one team member in particular who just couldn't adapt to the changes and improvements we put into the office. We exhausted all training options we had at the time, and had documented all crucial conversations and performance conversations well. But the time came when the team was too frustrated with working with the individual, and it was time to move on for the greater success of the office. Our Director of Operations let the individual go, and "allegedly" made one simple mistake. According to this individual, there was a remark made along the lines of, "You may enjoy some time off at this point" which was interpreted by the ex-employee as violating the venerated non-discrimination act protecting age, sex, race and religion. Big no-no. What followed was a lawsuit against us for over $150,000 (the employee's salary multiplied by the number of years left until retirement). Many depositions, full day meetings, expensive overtimes, testimonies and a $30,000 attorney bill resulted in the case being judged in favor of Infinity Dental Partners, but we saw first hand how a little HR situation can rock your world! Whether you keep it in house or you outsource HR, it's mandatory!

PRODUCTION DIVISION

Production division's goal is to ensure the office is in a healthy production and collection level throughout each month and is on track to hit their monthly goal. The primary role is to provide coaching support and strategize with offices that are falling short of daily goals and hitting bonus. Production division communicates with the treatment coordinator office to audit daily goal levels for each doctor and hygienist and ensure the levels are appropriate for the office and attainable.

Production division audits the number of days goals are met by reports in the middle of every month and at the end of the month. The report in the middle of the month allows production division to coach and support offices that are close to hitting bonus. Additionally, production goals are audited twice per year to ensure that growing offices' goals are appropriately raised.

CASE ACCEPTANCE DIVISION

Case Acceptance division ensures the case acceptance rate with new and existing patients is at a level that facilitates a healthy practice and increases growth, while keeping in line with hitting the break even point and the month bonus goal for the team. Case Acceptance division assists and coaches treatment coordinators and continually monitors their protocols and communication to ensure they help further create value for patients and assist in closing treatment. The percentage goal for case acceptance for our offices is 65% or above.

As you can see, as your group grows, the number of responsible managers to keep eyes on every aspect grows. Having done this for nine years, we can say that you will never become an owner until you create divisions of management. If you have to have your fingers in every aspect of your company and have to manage it yourself, you'll always be an operator but now your handpiece will be your offices. Setting up eight divisions of management truly lets you move from being an operator to a business owner.

Now let's talk about setting up a centralized command. As you can see in Diagram 1, you will have to coordinate a centralized command of bookkeepers who are coordinating satellite checking systems. You have to have a payroll process that expands to multiple offices and even multiple states. We experimented for several years to find the right flow that would facilitate good communication between teams and our bookkeepers, and good communication between our bookkeepers and our accountants. What we have found is that you will need one bookkeeper for every eight offices. Where in-house bookkeepers become absolutely imperative is if you ever get into a tight cash flow situation. At one point, we had outsourced bookkeeping and found that managing a cash flow crunch is very difficult when things are too automated. It's very difficult to manage vendor payments if you don't have your internal team handling the situation.

There was a period in 2012 where we got very deep in the hole and we were $598,000 behind on bills. It was a very scary period when we were getting letters from utility companies threatening to close down offices. We have so many memories as the leaders of our organization sweating it out on a Saturday night, trying to figure out how we were going to climb out, and what bills were going to be paid first. Having a couple good bookkeepers was part of the equation to maintain integrity with our doctors and our vendors.

When the going got tough, they were able to have conversations and set up payment plans, and manage every penny of the cash flow to prioritize the most important vendors. They simply created an art to the cash flow management. When the cash is great, that's less important. We know now that having good bookkeepers to keep an eye on and manage your cash flow is critical early on when the margins are tighter.

A quick overview of our satellite checking system: we have found that you have to set up a merchant service account with a local bank and set up satellite checking systems where checks can be scanned and sent directly to a central office. You're going to have cash coming in, you're going to have checks coming in, you're going to have credit card payments coming in, you're going to have insurance payments coming in. Ensuring that all sources are accounted for, tracked and put into an electronic format that can be managed makes everything easier. You'll never have people stuffing money into envelopes and mailing it to you. Everything needs to be put into an electronic traceable way as part of the pillars of fraud and embezzlement protection.

Finally, we want to talk about setting up a centralized accounts receivable person or team. For almost two years now, we have had a centralized AR person who provides two things for every office. First, they clean up the often long, overdue AR of new offices in a systematic way. Second, they provide coaching and training for existing team members on what works and what doesn't to ensure a small AR. That way, once the backlog is cleaned up, we have a system in place to make sure it never happens again. Very rarely have we seen an office that has a perfect AR, so there's almost always room for improvement.

Once you acquire a certain number of offices, you can justify having a centralized AR person because of economies of scale. The way we pay our AR person is on a salary because when you do AR, you're going to have evening calls, and you're going to have weekend calls, and you need somebody who has a hunger and a drive and is willing to work almost at all hours. Unfortunately, most people are at work during the day so a lot of the calls will not happen during the day. Putting that person on salary makes sure that they are taken care of on the understanding that they have to be flexible. We also give a performance-based bonus of 1% of their monthly collections so they're motivated to hit a higher level every month.

We have found that our doctors and our teams love having a centralized AR person because it brings cash flow into every office, from which doctors will get a percentage. It helps deal with hard patients who don't want to pay for the value the doctors create and takes some of the burden off of the team. For your group, it creates a wonderful cash flowing position that always pays for itself. From a cost justification analysis, we found you have to have between five and six offices to hire a full time AR person and support the economies of scale.

This chapter recounts the basic infrastructure and how to set the foundation of your management team. Again, eight divisions of management, a centralized command of bookkeepers and a centralized AR person is your basic core team. Obviously, that does not include your accountants, and it does not include your attorneys and other outside sources but will get you off and running from a management perspective.

We are going to dedicate an entire chapter to what we call our Education Facilitator, the final position in your management team, the person who is responsible for training and implementation of management modules to optimize your office.

5

DEVELOPING A
TRAINING SYSTEM

Why are training programs so critical? One of our doctors, Dr. Ralph Beadle of Catlettsburg, Kentucky, gave us one of our favorite quotes: "Inspiration without information leads to frustration." We had spent many years developing a great culture, taking classes on public speaking, throwing motivational summits, and really working hard to transform the lives of our team members and our doctors on a mental, emotional and spiritual level. Our goal was to bring the concept of life coaching into dentistry and create a culture centered around life transformation. The problem is that you can get somebody very inspired and give them a great mission and vision for the office, but if you're all context and no content, you're going to have a team that doesn't know what to do with all that inspiration. They may be motivated as all get-out, but have no pathway and no tools with which to grow.

That's when we realized we had to develop a training program to implement everything that we do in a scalable, efficient way that can be modulated, can train people in their positions and in management systems, and can be used to back reference when necessary. That's when we developed the concept for Infinity Dental University. Of course there's a story behind this, as you might suspect, which goes all the way back to 2004. I (Jared) was a first year dental student at the University of Michigan. While I could hold my own academically, I did not have the motivation at the time to attend class. I was not the type of learner who could sit there all day and retain information; It just wasn't my M.O. for learning!

With my background of starting a Dot.com in software development for two years prior to dental school, I went to the faculty and IT department at the University of Michigan School of Dentistry and told them I had a vision. I had a plan to record our lectures and automate access to them, so that if you missed class, you would have easy access to the information. iTunes and iPods were in their infancy, and the Cloud was yet to exist. So I led the development of three pilot studies to test how students in dental school learned best utilizing technology, and what system was most preferred. We did audio recordings, we did PowerPoint presentations with our audio recordings attached, and we did video. At the end of the year, we found that audio recordings were what students preferred, because of the portability. You could walk to class and listen to half of the lecture. You could even listen to a lecture while you were working out.

We developed an automatic program to record lectures at the touch of a button, and when the recording was finished, at the end the lecture, the file would be automatically uploaded to what we now call the Cloud. It then could be downloaded into iTunes and synced to your iPod. This was also before the iPhone ever came out.

The system worked incredibly well, and someone in the IT department had a contact with Apple, Inc. This was before Apple, Inc. was one of the largest companies in the world, but it was still a monster in the technology industry and had a lot of its focus, at the time, in education. So Apple flew a team in, evaluated our system, loved it, and we co-created what is now called iTunes U. iTunes U is an online portal for universities to upload all of their lectures and provide content access to the world and to their students. Now you can listen to nearly every lecture from all the great speakers in every university. iTunes U is presently in over 800 institutions around the world. I traveled the country, spoke on behalf of Apple at several education events, and was invited to participate in a think-tank session in Cupertino at Apple's headquarters with their senior vice-presidents, to help co-develop an aspect of the App Store when apps were first being created.

So I had this experience on the power of automation and the power of efficiently delivering information for the purpose of learning and growing. I also had the management experience of purchasing and running a group of practices, implementing the things that we did that we knew were successful in management, and testing them personally because we were practicing dentists. We combined the two, and created a recipe to revolutionize teaching for dentists and their teams.

We took our knowledge and our experience and we developed a studio with the highest grade production video cameras and recording equipment, and we began recording everything that we did in our offices that increased production, created a well-managed team, and created a wonderful patient experience.

Infinity Dental University fits into how people learn; by audio and by visual, not by reading in manuals and books. We've experimented over the years with two main ways to get our offices trained up: coaching and manuals. Coaching allows you to get deep into the root of conflict, deep into personality issues. A coach can get insights that a manual can't. Coaching provides a culture of growth and transformation, while manuals create a culture of micromanagement. The millennial generation is in a "We World" currently and has no interest in being run by manuals. While you do have to have manuals at times, and checklists in combination with auditing work very well, we have found that having a human element facilitates fantastic culture and you can't put a price on that. Our University has five elements: A series of training videos by the two of us setting the Context of the two-week training, a series of training videos by our Education Facilitator providing the Content and Implementation aspect, a library of supporting manuals and forms, live coaching sessions in the form of a group collaboration session and weekly personal business coaching sessions for the doctor and team leaders, and a series of accountability quizzes to measure the progress of the office.

We realized that if you're going to have successful long-term implementation and accountability, you have to have someone implement it. You can't rely solely on the team and a doctor to implement the training module by themselves. People inherently will not reach the highest level in our experience if they don't have a coach keeping them accountable. We all know as practicing dentists that we get really excited after attending a trade show, and we come back with some technology or some system that we want to implement, but we have so many things happening at once - all of the hats of management and seeing patients - that it becomes almost impossible to effectively implement something that affects every team member in the entire office. That's where a coach comes in. Our Education Facilitator guarantees implementation week by week, and holds everybody accountable.

Here's the schedule for our University: The team watches a Context Video and a separate Content and Implementation video at the beginning of every 2nd week. At first, we had the Facilitator watch it with them to be able to answer any questions at the first day of implementation, but we found that the real questions didn't come up until day 2 or 3 of implementation. Furthermore, we would have to schedule it during a production hour that way, which the doctors and the teams did not like because it lowered their chance at hitting bonus that month. So we switched it to their lunch hours on Monday with pre-recorded videos, and everyone was happier. We scheduled our coaching sessions every week with the doctor and the team leader, not the team, because they are the two greatest influencers in the office, and also the most stable personnel.

We created an Ask Me Anything collaborative live coaching session with the Education Facilitator so everyone was able to get on a group televideo session and share their experiences twice per month. We had a collaboration series in the past that allowed doctors and team members from specific departments to get together every quarter and share ideas and collaborate and talk about new things they wanted to implement. Again, we've found that any opportunity you can make to get group collaboration is powerful to the culture of your group. By combining a scalable learning environment that is based on training modules one at a time with an Education Facilitator who can work remotely, we've created a low overhead, efficient system to implement training.

Infinity Dental University gave us the answer to one of our biggest and most important struggles over the years; which is how to train and re-train our team members effectively and remotely. It allows us to take new information, new management models and systems that will come out even in future years and implement them on a massive scale so that everyone wins instantly!

6

CREATING AN
OUTSTANDING
CORPORATE CULTURE

As the CEO of your group practice, you're responsible for the *culture, vision and solvency* of your organization and as we have said before, culture trumps solvency. There are going to be times when you run into a scenario and have to decide, "Am I going to let culture guide this decision or solvency guide this decision?" Making the right decision and putting culture first in these scenarios is imperative as you grow a group. Here's why: once you develop a multiple practice group, your team members will talk between the offices. So if you screw one team member over saving a couple of bucks, it's a culture killer that will spread like wildfire to poison your organization. It doesn't matter if you have a zero tolerance policy for gossip, too. Ask us how we know.

There's a concept that you need to get very used to and that's called being *solid on your principles but flexible on your policies*. We know this goes against hardcore Fortune 500 corporate culture but we're not in that environment. You have to be flexible on the policies that you have in your handbook to make sure you're always putting culture first. The most common scenario we've run into is when there's a dispute over benefits or payroll; If you try to nickel and dime your team members, they will feel short-changed, and there is no amount of money that is worth the bad culture that you'll create if a team member has a vendetta against you.

For eight years, part of our successful model was to throw annual group summits for our group as a private, internal event. Here's what we found: if you want to effectively motivate someone, you have to create an emotional event that allows them to draw the line in the sand from where they have been up until that point and create a blank slate for their future. Our summits serve as the vessel to be able to rewrite the rules of how they're going to do business for their patients. You can't do this effectively in their normal comfort zone where they have all of their normal habits and routines and environment stacked on their shoulders. We found that getting team members out of their normal environment into a place that allows them to free up their minds provides an opportunity for massive growth both personally and towards something bigger when they're part of a group practice.

Annual group summits also provide some unique opportunities for training. We've had many group training events at our annual summits where trainers come in and do breakout sessions. This allows your offices to learn together, which in and of itself allows for group collaboration and team building. We do a lot of team building exercises in our summits to allow people to get love and connection with each other and again, feel like they're part of a bigger cause. Annual group summits also provide an opportunity to bring in speakers to teach business concepts and give team members that annual spark that they need with a little bit of fun mixed in.

Financially, you can count on an annual summit costing between $25,000 and $75,000 for a remote event for a group between 30 and 75 people. There are some ways to lower your cost and let's talk about that. One, if you make the event voluntary and not mandatory, as a company, you are not required to pay for the team member's travel pay, pay for their hourly wage while they travel, pay for their hourly wage while in the event, all of which inevitably leads to paying overtime for an event. That is one way to make it cost effective. The downside of that scenario is that by not making it mandatory, you are not going to get everybody at the event. This is where you have to weigh the culture versus solvency balance.

Let's dig a little deeper in how to create a winning culture for both team members and doctors. For team members, it really starts with giving them a bigger mission and vision. Years ago, we went down the path of getting into a model of promoting a vision of educating patients about the oral systemic connection. We centered everything of our vision around working with physicians, being more than just dentists and doing everything we could to integrate ourselves into the medical community. In reality, it wasn't as effective as we had hoped financially and took a lot of time and effort with little gain to the bottom line. However, we did see that it gave our team members a much bigger mission and vision and that was extremely valuable. When our hygienists and assistants felt like they were not just working on teeth and gums and were actually helping the overall health of a patient and were educating patients on larger body processes, it gave them a far bigger reason to come in to work motivated. It gave them far better conversations with patients and far better loyalty to our offices versus offices that had no model centered around the oral systemic connection.

Again, whether you choose the oral systemic connection or you choose another model, providing team members a mission and vision is paramount to create a winning culture. In a future chapter, we're going to discuss our one-day mission, vision, and value creation exercise that we do when we transition a new office. We spend an entire intensive day recreating a mission and vision with the team members and the doctor in an empowering process to start off the partnership.

We often use the term empowerment; this is one of the final aspects in creating a winning culture for team members. Empowerment is one of the three core values of our company. When you have empowered doctors and empowered team members, when you've given them the tools and then allow them the freedom to manage themselves, it creates a level of motivation that micromanagement just can't touch. In our organization, we promote empowerment as one of the most important guide posts for operation on a daily basis. We make sure that with every management decision and every conversation we have with a team member, we strive to make sure that they feel empowered as a result. Empowerment is really the foundation of self-motivation. To disempower is to demotivate.

With our doctors, we work very hard on instilling a mission and vision centered around a servant attitude. It would seem obvious - the idea of putting the patient first and centering your mentality as a group around patient centricity and a servant attitude - but in an increasingly competitive economy with decreased reimbursements in our industry, you certainly will find doctors who have lost faith in this principle. Every conversation that we have when managing our associates and our senior doctors is centered around doing the right thing, putting the patient first, no matter what. There is no amount of money that will justify not putting the patient first. As the CEOs of our organization, our job is to provide massive value and support for our doctors. The reality is they produce 70 to 80% of the income of your enterprise. That means they deserve 70 to 80% of your attention if you're a good business owner. That's why we spend so much time creating and focusing on what we call our brotherhood-sisterhood mentality.

Most solo practitioners are used to working and living on an island. Yes, they have colleagues in the area and they're part of their local district dental societies, but they ultimately are competing with the other doctors. Having practiced for the last decade, there's no doubt that there's an island mentality and there's also a craving for love and connection that is symbiotic and not competitive. Group practice provides an unbelievable opportunity for collaboration and creating a culture of inclusiveness.

To feed this system, what we have done is quarterly collaboration series with our doctors by getting everyone on Skype and WebEx with an outcome-based plan of how to spend an hour and share ideas, share what's working and what's not, and talk about a case or two. Call it our own little internal Seattle Study Club, but we see the power of taking a doctor off the island and making him or her feel like they're a part of something bigger with brothers-and sisters-in-arms.

As part of creating outstanding corporate culture centered around a servant attitude, it's imperative to have a plan to get involved in the community. We've had two primary ways that were both very successful in getting our doctors and their teams involved. First, our free dental days. Now we know it's been overplayed and every dentist has tried it, but there is a reason and when you have a group practice, you can take it to different levels. For several years, we did solo free dental days. But when you have a group practice, you can start doing it as a group and get more bang for your buck in terms of marketing.

There are two ways to do a successful free dental day. One is to advertise and allow everyone to show up in the parking lot, camping out if necessary, and to take them as time allows. Our first three annual free dental days we did it this way. It really creates a buzz and an energy that can be a lot of fun! We had porta-potties, barbecues, tents, and kids' activities in the parking lot to create a really unique environment that was more of a celebration than just another day at work. However, there are some downfalls that come with this scenario. One of the days that we did it in this fashion, it thunder-stormed for part of the day and became quite miserable because we didn't have a waiting room big enough to hold everybody. Although there were tents, we had 300 people in our parking lot at one of our offices. As you can imagine, that led to some pretty miserable conditions.

The other scenario is to do a lottery system and schedule your patients out as you would on a traditional day. There are advantages and disadvantages to this. It is far more controlled, less chaotic and more like a normal day to schedule a certain number of people per hour on a predetermined schedule. However, the disadvantage is that you do lose some of the energy and excitement and community bond that occurs by having a big group together. It really does just feel like a normal, average day at the office. So choose your own adventure. If you go the lottery route, the protocol that we use is to advertise the event four to six weeks prior. Give the patients a one week period where they have to come in, fill out a basic demographic ticket with their name, address, phone number, email, and chief concern. Then for one week they can stop by and submit it into a big pot. We do a drawing of a predetermined number of patients, based on the capacity and the number of doctors and team members working, and then call each of those patients to get them scheduled, while creating an alternative list for no shows.

Our other major community service program, which has really taken over free dental days in the last two years, is iSmile. We were the pilot group for a new program unlike anything dentistry had ever seen. Jay Riggs, the founder of Will Play For Food Foundation, developed a foundation with a vision of ending child hunger nationally using a tax write-off incentive program for businesses and communities to get involved. The greater picture is to unite small businesses to actually be the driving force at a local level of educating and providing meals for children by donating charitable meals.

The way it works in our offices is that we first create a launch event with our teams, centered around this unbelievable opportunity of involving dentistry and combating childhood hunger. There's an entire branding campaign in terms of wearing scrubs with iSmile logos, custom mission statement posters, banners, and just about everything you can imagine to create an identity around this daily community service event within your office. It's a hardcore branding campaign you sign up for! The skinny for the program is that for every patient visit in one of our offices, we donate 10 nutritious meals that are distributed by our zip code through the two largest food pantries in the country. Sounds expensive right? In reality, it is the corporate matching of Will Play For Food Foundation that makes it 10 donated meals with an overhead of $1. That's $1 per patient visit that's donated.

Furthermore, it's a charitable donation and is a wonderful tax write-off for your enterprise, especially when multiplied by multiple offices. When a patient comes to our office, there's a protocol that we take them through with iSmile in which we educate them and make them feel a part of this greater mission to combat child hunger. We let them know that we're donating meals to children in our community every time they visit. We have a graph and a meter, both for patients and for our offices as a whole, showing how many meals we've donated. We have done community events centered entirely around iSmile. We participated in one of the largest parades in one of our Michigan communities in which we had two floats centered around iSmile. We branded our floats to demonstrate to the community that when you visit one of our exclusive dental offices, we donate meals to children in our community as part of our greater mission to educate on child nutrition and help end child hunger. You want to talk about having a competitive edge and an incredible IIR opportunity? Everybody does free dental days, but nobody uses dentistry to combat child hunger.

Finally, a unique way that we developed an outstanding corporate culture was by developing a corporate coin based on our values and our mission (see Diagram 2). This is a concept seen in the military where each division of the military has a challenge coin symbolizing their division of the military, or their mission or tour of duty. As the story goes, if you're at a bar and somebody comes in and throws their coin on the table, if you don't throw your coin down because you forgot it, you have to buy them a drink. We created our own corporate coin because we have a brotherhood/sisterhood that is unbelievable and we wanted our doctors and our team members to have a daily reminder. We also learned this concept from the employees of the Ritz Carlton, as they have in their pockets a daily reminder of being part of something greater and of the values they stand for.

Our three principles on our coin - empowerment, purpose, and integrity - are guiding lights for our doctors and our team members, especially during tough times. Let's discuss a couple of examples. One of our doctors, who had our coin for over a year, had a daughter who was graduating from college, and they were on vacation together. They were having a heart to heart conversation about some of the challenges and the direction that she wanted to go in her career path. Our doctor told us that while sitting on a beach, having this heart to heart with his adult daughter, he pulled out the coin and they held it together and he said, "Is this decision you're making in your career in line with integrity for yourself and for your values? Is this decision in line with you feeling empowered and will it give you an empowering future? Is this decision in line with your greater purpose and what you want to accomplish in life?" And he said in mutual tears they made decisions together, and felt like they had a little token of guidance to help them, giving them insight together!

The other scenario involved an associate doctor who's been with us for six years and who is within a year of being able to purchase one of our offices. We have been coaching the doctor on leadership skills and integrating him into the decision process to get him ready to be a sole owner of the practice. One of the team members at his office created a scenario that forced our hand to have to terminate their employment. The doctor, after consulting with our divisions of management, took it upon himself to be the person to step up and have the crucial conversation and lead the discussion side by side with our HR department. He held the coin in his hand, with his hand in his pocket, while he had the discussion. He sent us an image (see Diagram 3) afterwards describing how he had one of the more difficult conversations he's had to have in his six years of practice, but felt confidence by having the coin in his hand knowing the principles we've taught and the culture he's a part of. That is priceless.

We're going to revisit our Due Diligence Checklist later in the book. A large part of why we almost lost everything in 2012 was because we didn't follow it properly, so it's importance must be emphasized.

7

CREATING AN
ACQUISITION TEAM

Why is an acquisition team so critical to the process of developing your own group practice? Because early on, it's all about time management. When you're practicing dentistry and seeing patients, focusing on providing a world-class experience and also an unbelievable crown prep, there is no way your mind can be off in entrepreneurship-land thinking about the doctors you have to talk to that day. You simply don't have time to effectively be a clinician and an entrepreneur without some help. We say this because we did it for many years. One of the things that makes us unique in the industry is that we built our group for an eight-year period while practicing clinical dentistry the entire time, so we have a very unique relationship with time management. Time management is everything.

Also, when you're doing dentistry and you don't have the time to call someone back until that evening or maybe the next day when you have a break in the schedule, you lose trust. Speed equals trust in the business world. Speed is the fastest way to instantly gain credibility and develop integrity with the relationships around you. What we have found in the past is that if you delay a response by even 24 to 36 hours, you instantly lose credibility. How can you preach that group practice provides efficiencies when it takes you a day to return a phone call? That's not efficient. Furthermore, the sheer number of steps and the required tracking and accountability can get very overwhelming if you do not have at least one individual keeping the process accountable for success.

Finally, having an acquisition team is in line with the industry standard. Dentists are used to the idea of brokers managing a process of acquisitions and it's too much of a pattern interrupt to have it go dentist to dentist. That's taking them out of their comfort zone and when they are dealing with selling their prized possession, their baby for the last 10 to 30 years, they take it very seriously and are not going to work with something too far out of their comfort zone.

In a related topic, an acquisition team also acts somewhat as a third party mediator. Let us explain. During the process of a transition and all the steps that come with evaluating an office, emotions can run high at times. When contracts get negotiated between attorneys representing both sides and there are disputes on the terms, things can get heated. It's great to have a quarterback mediating the facts and the agreements during that so that you don't damage the relationship. Real world example? We had courted practice Y for over six months in our evaluation process and had invested three personal visits with this doctor developing a relationship, and they attended two of our seminars. At the point when we were ready to look at contracts, we already had a very strong relationship. However, Doctor Y's attorneys had some issues with our contracts and sent a pretty heated email regarding one or two points. We got heated in return on some points that we thought were unreasonable, especially given our experience in the industry. Yet we had a quarterback who was able to calm down both parties, come up with a solution and move forward without damaging the relationship, and preserving a great partnership.

This leads us to the point that every doctor thinks his/her practice is worth more than it's actually worth. You have to remember that doctor has been in that office for 25, maybe 35 years and he has put everything into that practice. So naturally, you cannot blame him for thinking that his practice is worth 90% or even 100% of what it's collecting annually. This is why it is critical that you have a transition person trained in the methods of appraising practices.

Another critical element in creating an acquisition team is having the proper systems to guide the process of an acquisition and keep it organized. Over the years, it started with a single piece of paper essentially being emailed to the two of us with a demographic overview of the doctor and their office collections, their active patient count and their story. It has evolved into an incredibly efficient series of solutions that are easy to access and portable, and allow us to have all the information we need for making business decisions.

The first system that we worked with and mastered is called Basecamp. Basecamp is a powerful software solution that allows you to organize individual projects, keep all of their related documents and checklists in one place, and provide equal universal access to everyone involved. In addition, it can be taken with you everywhere you go. The reason you need a tool like this is that it keeps everyone on the same page and keeps everyone updated when managing multiple potential practices. Once you start talking to multiple practices that are at various points of the courting phase and the transition phase of owning practices, there are too many moving parts at once.

Furthermore, no two practices are ever closed in exactly the same way. The very nature of dental offices and how they are setup by different accountants and different attorneys with different debt structures necessitates custom agreements and custom deals to move the partnership forward. You need a centralized spot for all parties to access the information because your own accountants and attorneys will need to translate those custom deals into legal language.

You have to have a convenient portable solution on your smart phone in our experience. There will be a day that you will be able to hang up the hand piece and the white coat, but until then (unless you're already there), you're going to be doing a balance of clinical dentistry and your entrepreneurship opportunity. Having a solution on our smartphone even versus a laptop is critical because again, it allows you to respond to your acquisition team as the CEO quickly, which allows them to develop speed and trust with the perspective doctor.

It also allows you to have a checklist to keep the process moving forward that updates everyone. We found that it's critical when you have five to seven parties moving down a process to have a checklist system to make sure you're moving from A to Z and nobody is repeating a step and creating a state of unprofessionalism.

So how do we use it? Personally, we only use it on our smartphones. You can download the app from either the Apple Store or the Android Store. Basecamp allows you to create individual Basecamps which are individual projects per doctor (see Diagram 4). We set it up so that each doctor's first and last full name are our individual base camps so that when we open up Basecamp, we see a list of doctor names and the last time they were updated as our active client list. This allows us to click on a doctor name and pull up the next page. At the top of every Basecamp, we have found the best way to organize it is to put the town or city first, followed by the state, the contact information, and what specific deal you are working on with that doctor (see Diagram 5). For example, are you looking to purchase 100% of their office, are you looking at purchasing 50% of their office, or are you looking at a manage-to-own scenario. It tells you what users are on and allows you to control who has access to your Basecamp.

We don't use every aspect of Basecamp, but let's talk about those we consider critical. Let's talk about the Campfire section. When you click on the Campfire section, it's a continuous blog of all of the updates in conversation between all members on Basecamp (see Diagram 6). This allows us to be able to scroll back on conversations and gives us a feed of things happening at the moment in conversation style. There's a section in Basecamp called Message Board. We do not use Message Board, because in our experience, it gets too confusing with Campfire, and in our testing Campfire is the more effective solution.

The next critical piece is the To-Do List in Basecamp (see Diagram 7). Again, having a to-do list is critical but what's nice about Basecamp's To-Do List is it allows you to assign it to individual members in the acquisition team. Furthermore, it allows you to assign it to the calendar and give reminders of when those steps have a to-do date.

We then look at the Schedule aspect (see Diagram 8). What's nice about Basecamp's Schedule is that it allows all the members to know exactly the timeline of the to-dos in a visual format, and know when their by-whens are for those critical steps.

Finally, you have what is called the Docs and Files tab (see Diagram 9). Just like many other cloud-based document storage solutions out there, this gives you a centralized area to upload all of the related documents along the course of the transition, which again is critical on creating efficiencies. This alone makes Basecamp worth its while. The system we used prior to finding a portable online document system specific to the transition team was essentially using email and folders on computers that were not all connected. If somebody needs to see the proposal for Doctor X, I know that we can pull out our smart phone and they'll have it within 15 seconds, emailed to them directly from Basecamp.

Another system that's critical in the early stages of the development of your acquisition team and the process of courting a doctor is utilizing a call center. Now picture this: you're a clinical dentist and you are at your office doing a crown prep on a complicated patient, and all of a sudden you get a phone call, and then you get another phone call, and then you get another phone call. Before you know it, you have missed four phone calls that you felt ringing in your pocket and they were all potential doctors who wanted to be part of your group. This is what we have experienced, and this is why you must have a call center.

There will be a time and a day when your group will be large enough to justify a full-time employee to answer these calls. We even investigated the possibility of having your existing front desk personnel or team members answer calls for the business end, but we have found this is the best solution until that point. The problem with having an existing team member in your office answer calls for your business group is that it gets confusing and it also looks unprofessional. The identity that you are trying to create here is one of certainty, establishment and professionalism.

We have investigated and used several call centers in the past, and the one that we settled on is called Answer Connect. Answer Connect had one of the highest ratings on surveys for a quality product and service and provides an affordable solution to getting started for less $1500 annually (see Diagram 10).

So you have your communication system established, you have a call center to create speed and trust, and you've created an acquisition team. Now let's talk about the steps that the acquisition team needs to do, in our experience, to court a doctor and take them from first point of contact to transitioning them into your group.

There are eight steps in our acquisition team checklist. So you're probably wondering why eight steps, why not just get their profit and loss statements, think of a good price and then move forward? Well, you cannot go on a date and then get married the next day. You have to develop rapport, you have to develop certainty. You have to develop the relationship to be able to get to the final step which is closing. Research shows that there is a minimal number of times that a person must see or hear about a product and that number is at least five times. So we created eight to go above and beyond, to be thorough and more importantly, to develop that relationship.

The first step is a 30-minute phone conversation between the doctor and one of our acquisition team members. This is not a conversation that is with you, doctor to the doctor. Again, this is with your acquisition team acting as a third party. This conversation is designed to give us a 30,000 foot perspective overview of that doctor's practice and answer any questions that they have about the opportunity and about your organization. We found in the past that this 30-minute conversation can actually weed out good and bad practices. This conversation is the opportunity to discuss philosophies and see if they match or if they don't. It gives the opportunity to talk about the doctor's office location, about their values, and about their goals.

Step two is for the acquisition team to email you a summary of that 30-minute conversation (see Diagram 11). As you can see, there are some basic questions that are answered as a part of that 30-minute conversation to make sure it's productive and provide us some of the critical information to move forward. Your acquisition team may not know if it's a good fit at first, and this is one area where you need to provide your expertise if you're going to move forward.

The third step at that point, if you green-light an office, is for your acquisition team to schedule a 15 to 20-minute phone conversation for you to communicate directly with the doctor, doc to doc. This is doctor selling to doctor and the relationship is very different. This isn't a used car sale, this isn't something you're buying online with Amazon, this is a doctor selling their legacy to another doctor and it requires, in our experience, early-on skin-in-the-game in terms of the time spent in this process on your part. This 15 to 20-minute phone conversation is designed for the two of you to talk to one another about the possible acquisition of their practice. This is the opportunity for you to discuss philosophy. This is the opportunity for you to discuss standard of care. This is an opportunity for you to alleviate their fear of transition and is critical to developing an early culture or integrating this doctor into the culture that your group stands for. After this phone conversation, you will give your acquisition team either the red light to stop, or the green light that you would like to continue moving forward with this practice and this doctor.

Step four is for your acquisition team is to gather documents for the practice evaluation. In this step, your acquisition team is going to have the doctor gather some basic documents needed to evaluate their practice, such as their last two years of financial statements, their W2s for the last year, a production report for the last year, and our 12 page questionnaire. Gathering documents and completing the questionnaires takes about two hours of their time and is a selling point so that they understand this doesn't take weeks. The questionnaire is extremely thorough and really lets you take a deeper dive into the dynamics of their practice. It allows you to look at how many team members they have, what their payroll is, how many hours they work, a summary of their benefits, their paid vacation hours, their number of years working at the practice, their recent purchases of equipment, the age of some of their equipment, etc. Again, this allows you to get an in-depth view of their office and gives you more information to move forward. It also helps you when you come to a purchase price for the practice. For instance, you may find that in their profit and loss statement their Education budget is through-the-roof, but the reality is that in the questionnaire, you identified that they used a transition consultant in the past, but had categorized it as Education. This will help you with getting insight into the actual cash flow of the practice. Once those documents are gathered, the acquisition team forwards the information to your accounting team to discuss an appropriate purchase price based on all the information gathered, the demographics of the office and the terms in which you want to evaluate an office.

Step five is to present the practice evaluation and the terms of sale. This step, which takes place up to two weeks after the documents are gathered, is a one and a half hour meeting via WebEx or GoToMeeting to review the practice evaluation and review the findings of their practice (see Diagram 12). This practice proposal is in presentation form and is extremely thorough in terms of showing a doctor what their options are in the market, and what the numbers look like in terms of profitability of sale. It is geared towards not just showing them how the transition can provide them financial value, but also emotional value, and how it fits into their life plan.

Step six is a 30 to 90-minute phone call one week after the purchase proposal presentation. The accountants and attorneys of that doctor will be looking at the proposal as part of the practice evaluation, but we have found that many questions come up even at the doctor level after the purchase proposal presentation. We have found a separate phone call where we can answer any questions about our company and how this relationship will work is critical, and have developed an FAQ from the compilation of several hundred conversations over the years to help with the process.

Step seven may be the most important step of all. As we mentioned earlier, a doctor is buying you and your culture and the relationship as much as they are selling their practice. This is where you're going to want to have some kind of summit or seminar where the doctors come to you. The reason why you want them to come to you is because it is going to show their level of commitment to find out more about you and to find their level of commitment to sell their office. Another reason why you want to have this seminar is because you want to explain to the doctor what is in it for the team, what is in it for the doctor's patients and what is in it for him or her. This is where you can go into detail about the patient experience that they're going to be seeing. You can go into detail about what is going to happen with the team. You could pre-warn the doctor about certain questions that may arise from his/her team members. You can pre-warn the doctor about the transition of the patients and what those questions will be. And more importantly, it starts establishing that love and connection that you need to purchase his or her office.

Step eight begins with an agreement to move forward and a Letter of Intent. A letter of intent, while not a legal binding agreement, puts everyone's signatures on a page that says, "We agree to a purchase price and we're ready to take the next steps to get legal documents prepared and executed." Things can still change at this point, especially during the due diligence of the office, but we've found there is something emotional about putting your signature down that creates a sense of moving forward and a letter of intent says we're not wasting our time here.

The final step is a massive coordination of team members toward the goal of acquisition. A transition requires attorneys on both sides, accountants on both sides, both selling and buying doctor, the buying doctor's transition team and the selling doctor's clinical team to help set that office up for a smooth transition. All of that coordination needs to be identified and spelled out to create certainty before a closing day is set. In our experience, doctors like to know what happens on day one before day one happens. So it's critical to spell out the transition process with all parties involved.

Now let's talk about the Due Diligence Checklist. This is another eight-step checklist that is mandatory for your acquisition team to quarterback for a successful transition.

First, you need to have an in-depth financial review meeting with your accountant and the doctor and their accountant. Your acquisition team is going to supply all tax related documents, tax returns, the letter of intent, and a cash flow analysis, and provide all contact information of the selling doctor so that they can help create a purchase price or a practice evaluation. You are going to schedule a financial review meeting with your accountant and their accountant, and it's mandatory for the doctor to attend. The reason we do this first checklist item in our due diligence is that accountants and attorneys can create barriers in the process. It has been our experience that most accountants who work for dentists don't understand transitions, and they only understand basic accounting of the daily running of a practice. They don't understand the financial ramifications of doing a transition the right way or the wrong way. They don't understand how to manage the capital gains of a bank-financed transition versus the increased income tax bracket of an owner-financed model. We have found that hitting it hard and hitting it upfront with both accountants on the line creates certainty for the doctor, and gets a lot of those FAQs answered right out of the gate.

The second due diligence checklist item is a walkthrough of the office. You must schedule an office walkthrough either physically or with a video camera. We found that certainly the ideal, if you're going to purchase a million dollar company, is to go visit the office and go do a walkthrough yourself. While it's okay to have a team member there, this is ideally done outside of business hours to protect the doctor. A lot of doctors aren't ready to tell their team members that they are ready to sell or enter into a partnership, and it can foster internal turmoil and employee turnover if this information gets out, because transition can equal uncertainty for some team members. We are very careful to protect this process and to protect the doctor to help create a smooth transition with the team. Doing an initial video walkthrough of an office can be valuable if you have a doctor who is nervous about having someone come see the office, because he has not shared his intention with the staff or community. The doctor can send a video walkthrough with a Flip video camera very efficiently and inexpensively. It will allow you to oversee if this is actually an office that you want to purchase from a physical standpoint.

The third step in our due diligence checklist, after a letter of intent is signed, is to have your attorney get access to all of the financial information and update your legal documents with all of the appropriate information; i.e., demographics, dates, purchase price and terms. In our experience, this step costs between $5,000 and $10,000 and generally takes two to three weeks of time. This is also the step where you choose a closing date that can be put in the contract. The great news is this gives a light at the end of the tunnel because it puts a definitive date to when this is going to get done, as it is coordinated around the legal closing date of the closing documents. After your attorney updates the contract specific to this practice acquisition, they send those contracts to the selling doctor's attorneys and we give them a specific "by-when" of when we expect any feedback. If you do not put a by-when at this critical step, you are going to be relying on the selling doctor's attorney's schedule and it can really slow down the momentum of the process.

The fourth step is to have an on-sight equipment analysis and a fee schedule report done. We use our products and services vendor to analyze the equipment and also provide a fee schedule report. Providing a fee schedule report shows us where they are and where there are some potential immediate increased revenues. We've been amazed over the years what little attention this critical element has received from practices and how low some practices have priced certain procedures. As a whole, we try to keep our fee schedule at the 60th percentile, in the belief that we are almost in the exact middle, but believe our services deserve to be slightly above the mean for the surrounding 10 mile radius in terms of fees. Doing an on-sight equipment analysis will save your butt and here is why. We have had several transitions where we purchased an office and on day one, something wasn't working properly, the computers were outdated, the server needed to be replaced or a chair was down, and it wasn't disclosed. You'll find the most common update needing to be done will be the computers and network. We have seen this so many times that we actually generally build this into the budget. It seems to be one of the missing links that's left out in terms of updating the technology of an office. Doctors tend to think if it works well enough, they don't need to update it, but in reality, to do some of the software programs and to stay in HIPAA compliance, you generally need a beefier system than most doctors think.

This leads into our fifth due diligence checklist step, which is to have an IT analysis done of their software, and to do an audit for compliance. We have a software solution that we install called Dental Information Tracking System that we co-created with our accountant. We are going to get into further detail in future chapters, but as part of our due diligence, we get that scheduled for installation.

The seventh step is a pre-closing business office setup checklist item. As we identified, you are going to setup a centralized command that is going to go through their own specific checklist of steps that have to happen prior to closing date. For example, they're going to have to contact your centralized banking. They're going to set up an EIN number, and they're going to set up checking accounts and remote checking scanners. This all has to happen no later than four weeks prior to the closing date for a smooth transition.

The final step on the Due Diligence Checklist is actually scheduling and attending an on-sight closing visit or a remote closing event through DocuSign. In our early years, we found it necessary to do an on-sight closing event. However, in recent transitions, we found the efficiency of using DocuSign is favored by both selling and buying parties. The beauty behind DocuSign is it's easy to instantly sign all related documents and share with all parties involved, including the attorneys and the accountants, at the click of a button. Furthermore, you have a digital record on the Cloud so that in the event of fire or any related event, you know that those sacred documents which are the connection between being a solo practitioner and a multi-millionaire entrepreneur are protected. It's also a lot easier to use your electronic documents to transfer to your electric storage area or App whether that be Dropbox or Google Drive.

8

MARKETING
FOR PRACTICES

Location is everything. The age-old real estate phrase holds true for finding additional practices. As you venture out and start looking for your practice, you have to start with the right plan based on location and then reverse-engineer it. We made the mistake, in our second phase of growth, of marketing too broadly and having practices too spread out geographically. You'll learn in this chapter why that can be to your detriment and how to avoid that. Here's the big warning we can't reiterate or emphasize enough: Don't get tempted by the huge market outside of your local area and start marketing like crazy 100, 200, 300 miles away. Keep it close, build your systems, then expand.

Our experiences gave us wisdom which we utilized to create a better plan. We created the Cluster Rule. The Cluster Rule is a concept of only purchasing dental practices within a 30-mile radius of each other. Let's go into the key benefits of the cluster rule. First, it creates freedom for you right off the bat. And isn't that a big reason you are interested in all of this? If you can find several practices close to your existing primary practice, it will be the fastest way for you to retire personally. If your goals are to become the owner of a large group, your time and attention will eventually mandate 100% of your time. And quite honestly, it's very exciting to see the light at the end of the tunnel when you know you can hang up the hand piece and the clinical coat. But the starting point to make that happen is radical common sense: you must create a local cluster around your surrounding practice. Your first five practices should be within 30 miles of your existing office, ideally. What that allows you to do is bring in your replacement right off the bat.

The most important benefit of The Cluster Rule pertains entirely to associates. Unless you plan on retiring immediately upon transition, or you're growing your office at more than 30% annually, it's very difficult to bring in a full-time associate and provide them the production that they need to sustain themselves and also keep enough profit in your pocket to sustain your lifestyle. Having two or three offices within short driving distances of each other allows you to offer an associate full-time employment and split their time between two or three offices. They can practice two days per week in office A and two days per week in office B, so that way you can offer them four full days. We have very rarely found an associate looking to settle down on two days per week. It instantly gives you a competitive advantage over every solo practice in town.

Another key benefit of following The Cluster Rule is that it allows you to create an anchor training office (which we call our flagship office) for the additional satellites. It's critical that you aim to make your first office in a new area an anchor training office. It should not be an office doing anything less than $800,000 in collections annually. It needs to be a more substantial office. It's not until you get to office two, three, or four that you can dive into offices in the $300,000 to $800,000 annual collection range. There is not enough stability or growth potential to justify the time and finances required to make a smaller office a training center. When you have a training center created within your anchor office, the moment a satellite office joins your cluster you will enroll the anchor team to become training facilitators for the new team members. This model does a few great things for your organization: 1) It gets your training team in your anchor office very excited, and gives them the sense of growth and contribution, 2) It provides variety for those team members and their daily routine, 3) It provides them additional income at the time of training. We pay the training team members an additional $5 per hour above their existing hourly wage. We generally have a satellite team member shadow them for a half-day session. This collaborative, mentor-type relationship also helps promote a culture of education and support amongst your cluster group. There's no better way than on-site shadowing and training to learn the systems of your group, and it really falls in line with one of the most effective ways to quickly train a new team member. Think of it as the tell-show-do methodology in person on a local level.

Another key benefit of The Cluster Rule is bang for your buck by providing the ability to manage several offices at once. If you have a local cluster hundreds of miles away from your central command and you have to do an office visit, you can kill several birds with one stone by reducing your overhead in terms of flight and hotel costs, having an office manager visit several offices on one trip. The alternative - sending them all over the country or all over the state one office at a time - is inefficient and expensive.

Finally, a key benefit of The Cluster Rule is sharing team members and ensuring coverage when a team member is sick or on vacation. Again, it goes back to creating a culture of helping each other. It requires coordination and communication with team leaders and your corporate management team, but it is so beneficial when, for example, an assistant is sick or a hygienist is sick, and you can contact the other satellites of your cluster, find out what their capacity is for the day and if they have the availability to share a team member. Normally, within one hour you have same day coverage. It's almost impossible in any other model, even with a temp agency, to get same day coverage for someone who's sick or someone who has to quickly leave the office. With our organization, it goes in line with the culture that we create which is one of support and one of team mentality.

So now that you know what our successful model is, a model that we have tested time and time again, let's discuss what type of practice to look for. First of all, let's talk about how to quickly evaluate an office's numbers in less than five minutes to discover its potential. We know that you never buy an office on potential, and that you only buy on what its existing profit, collections, overhead, etc. are. But there is a way to look at an office that is just radical common sense, and it allows you to see where the internal growth possibilities are. It's entirely centered around comparing what their active patient count is compared to their annual collections.

First, we calculate the value of a single patient. Management companies have calculated this number to be an average of all of the patients who require no treatment against all of the patients that require extensive treatment. They have come up with an industry standard that one active patient is equivalent in value to the sum of one crown, one core build-up, one set of bitewings, one exam and one prophy per year. The average added up will be different for every office, in every area, based on fee schedule, but you can calculate that it will be generally somewhere in the range of $1200-$1500 per patient. So if you know the value of one active patient is $1500 and you know office A has 2,000 active patients, you multiply the two, and the lost potential is the difference between that calculation and what their annual collection is. So again, that office with 2,000 active patients should be producing $3 million a year if at 100% optimized level.

Now obviously, no office will ever achieve this number and it's a pipe-dream to think that you ever will, but that's not the point. If that office with 2,000 active patients is only doing $600,000, we know they have a capacity to do $2.4 million more from just what's inside their practice with no external marketing. Now if that office with 2,000 active patients was doing $2.2 million annually, making the lost potential only $800,000, there would be far less room to tap into what already exists in the office. It's also an indicator that an office may be extremely specialized in full-mouth restorations and cosmetic dentistry, which gives you an indicator that the dentistry has likely already been done in all the existing patients. All things being equal, if you had office A and office B and they both had 2,000 active patients - where one was doing $600,000 and one was doing $2.2 million annually - we would buy the $600,000 office without question. There's just more potential to tap into, and we would be terrified of the $2.2 million office, because it's all used up or they're too specialized.

Let's go over a real world example we experienced. We had an office and a doctor C that we were looking at in 2011. We loved the doctor, we connected so incredibly well and developed a great relationship as we were courting each other. The doctor was doing $1.8 million annually in collections and was taking home $1 million cash in his pocket every year. He had an unbelievable practice, a brand-new building, and newer equipment, so it seemed like a home-run, until we dived into the numbers. The numbers tell us everything. He had 900 active patients. He was doing more than 100% of what his equivalent lost potential would be. With an office doing $1.8 million in annual collections, if you're looking at a bread-and-butter practice, he should have had several thousand active patients. So we looked at the 900 active patients and it immediately gave us direction on where the conversation should go. What we found is that the type of dentistry that he did was essentially full-mouth veneers, full-mouth reconstruction. He had a radio program in the area and was the go-to guy in his city to get a full set of veneers. And he was charging $25,000 to $40,000 per patient and had dozens of these patients every year going into his practice. The problem was, we would have had to rely on him and his reputation as an individual - that type of practice is so specific to the doctor, so specific to the doctor's reputation that when that doctor retires that marketing strategy retires with them. No associate can just come in and pick it up doing the same type of dentistry with the same numbers; it took years to get there. The other problem was that the majority of those 900 active patients were already in full-mouth restorations and had all the dentistry done. They were in hygiene maintenance mode at that point. In fact, to make things worse, we would have been carrying over the previous dentist's warranty on their dentistry if a veneer popped off or a crown broke. It was actually the worst possible practice to buy and was a ticking time bomb; thank God we walked away. And we'll be the first to tell you, it stings to walk away from an office with so little overhead and such a large take-home income. But again, until you analyze the numbers and understand this equation and understand what the numbers tell you, you don't know what you don't know.

The ideal practices to purchase if you're going to set up a multi-office group are bread-and-butter general dentist offices. Stay away from over-specialized practices. Those doctors are too hard to replace, it takes too many years of training and we would highly recommend staying away unless they plan on being onboard for five to ten years in a great contract. If that doctor is planning on leaving in less than two years, walk away from the practice. In our experience, it would be way too hard and you would lose too much money transitioning an associate who's not at that skill level. We know that this is counter-intuitive to what the progress of dentistry as an industry should be, and what we want for ourselves and the way we practice clinical dentistry, but you have to get yourself out of that mindset. You're an entrepreneur owning and managing a group of offices and doctors. Setting the foundation right is everything.

Now let's talk about location. In our experience, it's best to find offices within 45 minutes of a major metropolitan area, on a street that has 30,000 plus traffic flow per day, and where you're able to have a lit up sign at night that's large and can be set perpendicular to the road. However, most importantly, and in fact the over riding factor, comes down to one thing and one thing only: Would an associate live there? Quite honestly, this is everything, because as a group practice owner, one of your number one headaches and one of your most important factors for success is associate placement. If the practice is in an area where an associate would not want to live, you will have such a difficult time finding an associate doctor to replace the existing doctor or to add to the practice as you grow that it can become a nightmare. How bad? To the degree that you would have to prepare yourself to be the covering doctor for extensive periods. Let's look at a real world example. We bought an office in Punxsutawney, Pennsylvania. We bought the office on the plan of the doctor retiring two years after we signed on the dotted line. We knew it would be a struggle getting a doctor into an area like Punxsutawney, Pennsylvania based on the distance from a major metropolitan area and based on the demographics of that area. But in our naïve way, we still moved forward and proceeded in literally a 23-month venture of trying to find a doctor to move to and work full-time in Punxsutawney, Pennsylvania. We found doctors who were interested in joining our organization and believed what we stood for and loved the opportunity and the growth potential, but when they would go and visit the office, the number one thing we heard, and the reason we got so many "no, thank-you's," was the location. It had nothing to do with the team nor the practice nor the parent company managing them; it had everything to do with the fact that they could not ever see themselves living there, that their spouses would not be happy, and that it just wasn't going to fit in to their life.

The reality is that the future generation of dentists is the millennial generation, and the millennial generation is becoming more and more difficult to convince to live in rural small-town areas. Rural, small town areas have not caught up to metropolitan areas in terms of providing the lifestyle and the amenities that the millennial generation of dentists desires. It's too bad that all dental schools are in urban areas and dental students get used to that life! Of course, there are exceptions to the rule and of course, you will eventually find someone, but be prepared for a long struggle with a lot of lost potential associates if you choose an area that's not desirable for an associate to habitate long term.

Finally, let's talk about personality tests. In the beginning, we'd wing it and our way of evaluating a doctor was based on spending time with the doctor, taking them out to dinner, getting to know each other, developing rapport, and having a gut instinct of whether they're great or they're not, that we liked them or we didn't. We had no measurable way to really dig into their personality and see what worked and what didn't. So we decided to go the route of utilizing personality tests. Here are some examples of ones that we've used in the past: Myers Briggs assessment, DiSC tests, and Caliper Corp assessments.

You'll find that some of the personality tests are expensive and can cost a few hundred dollars upfront. When you're interviewing multiple associates, that can get expensive. But we learned our lesson on how important they are, and it only took one time. In our Ohio office, office D, we had been a year and a half into owning the practice, it was a double doctor team and they were ready to start transitioning out. So we adhered to our standard plan and opened up our associate placement relationships for that office, and found a local doc who was seemingly a perfect fit. He was from the area, he was a farmer, he wanted to settle down near the same area where the office was; it seemed like a dream situation for everybody. We didn't use any kind of personality test at the time. We just met him and interviewed him. He seemed like a great guy, and seemed to match our philosophies in clinical dentistry, so we onboarded him into the practice. Within one month, half of the team wanted to quit. His ability to communicate with team members was one of the worst we had ever seen or heard of. The senior doctors themselves gave us specific examples of things that he would say to team members that demonstrated his inability to communicate and manage basic relationships. We ended up having to let the doctor go, but it cost us one team member and many patients because they were turned off by their experience with the doctor. We learned our lesson and now have associate doctors do personality tests to make sure we can potentially have a compatible working relationship.

So how do you find practices? We want to talk about a successful marketing technique that we have mastered. We dabbled into a little bit of everything, measured what gave the greatest return and put our focus there. Our number one most successful marketing technique is very simple. It's a custom letter (see Diagram 13). As you can see, it's short, it's sweet and it's concise, but it targets the problems that doctors face on a daily basis. It targets the pain that they feel and articulates that a transition with us can be the escape from that pain. There are a couple of key points about this letter. The first key to success is that it comes from a dentist. There again is the doctor-to-doctor connection, where there's a different trust level. In terms of getting through the gate keeper, a letter from a dentist to a dentist will have a better chance of not getting thrown out.

The second key is that it's handwritten on the outside of the envelope. This isn't mass printed. We actually hire a person to hand-write the outside of every envelope. Our tests have found a significant increase in call rate by handwriting the envelope, because envelopes that are presented that way are more personalized, and are a pattern-interrupt against the standard type print.

The third key to success is that we put on the outside of the envelope that it's confidential for the doctor. This alone will potentially lower the chance of the gatekeeper throwing it away, and adds a tone of seriousness to the letter.

The fourth key to success is that getting a letter in a handwritten envelope in the mail in and of itself is a pattern-interrupt to how dentist are marketed. Dentists are used to getting bombarded with direct mailers. They're used to getting faxes and emails everyday of things being marketed to them. A handwritten letter is an interrupt to the standard way of marketing to a dentist and in and of itself increases the chances of being opened.

The final unique attribute, that we found interesting, is that because it has a higher chance of getting past the gatekeeper, being opened up and read, doctors will tend to hang on to it. We have found that it actually becomes a career milestone event, emotionally, when a doctor transitions. We've actually had three doctors specifically tell us that they looked back and remembered that moment that they received a letter from Infinity Dental, and how opening that letter was a milestone that changed their life forever. It's not on the same level as remembering where you were when the J.F.K. assassination occurred, but it's certainly an emotional milestone, and part of the story that doctors look back on with a smile.

9

ONBOARDING
AND COURTING
PROSPECTIVE
DOCTORS

After the initial marketing has captured the interest of a perspective doctor, we have found there's a very specific process that increases your chances of onboarding them with your vision and motivating them to sell.

You want to have multiple touch points when you're courting doctors. It's very easy for the day-to-day routine to get in the way of the doctor with whom you are communicating. For this reason, we have created what we call our "shock and awe" package. Our shock and awe package does two things: 1) It provides a massive amount of information upfront, designed to show the massive value created by joining our organization, 2) It is designed to facilitate multiple touch points over a several week period so that you are always in the forefront of the doctor's mind, and they never get lost in the system. In our experience, it's very easy for weeks to go by with no contact as you're waiting for accountants to talk, and as you're waiting for doctors to set up appointments with their attorneys. In the age of marketing bombardment and overload, you want to make sure you are staying in the forefront of their minds.

So let's discuss the contents of the "shock and awe" package. First, it contains a letter from our transition team that discusses the context and the content of the package. It also includes a call-to-action plan to show doctors what to do next, which is a 30-minute phone call conversation to follow-up the "shock and awe" package.

Tony Robbins created a seven-step plan of sales, and it all begins with rapport. If you're going to influence someone, you have to develop great rapport, and rapport starts with great connection. So we include a heartfelt autobiography. When we wrote our autobiographies, they were different than the ones we wrote for our website as clinical practitioners. This is not going to patients. This is going to other doctors. You have to find out how to connect with them and how to be relatable. We talk about our families, and we talk about our history in a way that puts out a bigger vision for the doctors instantly.

The next white paper that we include is called the *History and Vision for the Future* and it's about our grassroots movement to change dentistry. This document gets to the heart of the culture of our organization and our philosophy as entrepreneurs. The reality right now is that some large D.S.Os are damaging the reputation of dentistry. We demonstrate that we are willing to stand up for what's right and stand up for putting the patient first and preserving the integrity of dentistry, and have found that doctors will stand behind us for this cause. We have found that our culture sells as much as our content does. Yes, we have systems, but systems don't lead to massive emotion.

After explaining our culture and our mission as an organization, we want to give the doctor a roadmap of what is to come. So we create a document called *The*

Process in Which we Evaluate Each Other. This is a step-by-step roadmap so the doctor knows what's to come and where they are right now. As mentioned in the previous chapter, this includes the 30-minute phone conversation. It also involves filling out a 12-page questionnaire, gathering documents for practice evaluation, presenting the practice evaluation and terms of purchase, a follow-up phone conversation, attending our doctor information summit, signing a letter of intent, and starting to implement the transition stage.

The next white paper we include is entitled *Selling Your Practice To An Associate.* This document challenges the traditional model of dental transitions. There are some major problems that arise in traditional transitioning to an associate as a solo practitioner. For example, you generally have to give up chair time in order to provide enough dentistry for an associate to come in full time. Are you ready to sacrifice your income? Do you have enough capacity to keep them for more than three to six months? We know very well that when an associate comes in, there is generally a nine to twelve-month point where an associate will hit a wall as they use up all of the dentistry that created the original scheduling surplus. It gives the illusion that there was always enough dentistry there, when in reality, you just needed some help to get caught up. This creates a problem if the selling doctor is planning on staying on for a longer period.

Our model, based on The Cluster Rule, allows us to bring in an associate at a lower capacity and build them up to maximum capacity utilizing the power of multiple practices to maintain a full schedule on day one.

The next white paper gets into the meat of our organization; It's called *What Infinity Dental Brings to the Table*. This is an overview to show them exactly what services are provided by our organization, and how they're implemented. It really gets down to the nitty-gritty details. The majority of dentists will find this to be one of the most critical documents in the "shock and awe" package, because it's very thorough and really gives them a picture of what to expect.

We then include a white paper called *What Our Dentists Have to Say About Infinity Dental Partners*. We created a book in 2013 called *A Cup of Coffee with 12 Leading Dentists in the United States*, which was a series of biographies of our top 12 dentists at the time, and it also included a section on what they get out of being a part of group practice and a part of Infinity Dental. This white paper takes specific quotes from our existing doctors and specific testimonials to support their decision to join us. This is very powerful as it shows other doctors edifying the transition to group practice and testifying to the benefits.

Finally, our last white paper is a description of our group practice program. We created a program unlike anything on the market, to allow solo practitioners to fast-track building and owning their own group practice. If you're reading this book, you obviously understand the excitement that this provides. What you may not know is that we have created infrastructure to help you do it so it's not all on your shoulders. It took eight years, over $1.2 million invested into education, and a plethora of mistakes to get where we are today. We built the program around the understanding that if somebody had given us a roadmap and helped us in partnership, we would be much further ahead today, and would have avoided so many pitfalls. This document hones in on the hope for a greater future and shows practitioners that by joining our group, they can get on a pathway that they may never have known existed.

We had a meeting with several senior executives at one of the largest dental supply companies in the world in February 2016, and they made it very clear to us that multiple practice ownership is the hottest thing in dentistry for the next three to five years. We have a model that allows you to be a part of that market, now.

The other critical element to onboarding and courting prospective doctors is actually meeting them in person. This requires going to their office, meeting over dinner, going out to lunch, etc. If you have existing relationships with doctors in your area, we implore you to spend as much face time with them as possible, because that is how you effectively transfer vision and transfer hope for a greater future. We have found that the most effective way to emotionally connect with a prospect is a doctor-to-doctor information seminar. Having done these seminars for three years, more than several dozen times, we have figured out the right equation to make it work (See Diagram 14 for reference).

Additionally, we have found that if you use the steps that we are going to talk about, it is very possible to have a 100% closing rate. So what are some key points? First, keep it small and intimate. We have found that three to six doctors is the maximum number you should be looking for. If you go beyond six doctors, you start losing the personal touch. Two, realize that you're investing in relationship capital. The time you spend over lunch together is actually one of the most important hours of your day. That's where you get the love and connection, that's where you share stories with each other, that's where you talk about family, that's where they start feeling like they are part of your culture. Three, plan on a full day. There is no way you are going to be able to set the context and deliver the information on what to expect in anything less than a seven-hour presentation. Yes, it can be done, and we have done a combination of half-day and one-and-a-half-day infor-mation seminars, but our experiences, based on the presentation you can reference in Diagram 14, is that it's a seven-hour presentation. You'll see that the first half of the day up until lunch is set on delivering the context and the mission and the vision you have, followed by the company infrastructure. People aren't necessarily buying your systems, they're buying you. They're buying what you stand for. They are buying the "why." When somebody is selling their legacy and the baby that they built for 30 years, you'll find that preserving their legacy is equally important to the cash they'll get in their pocket. We've actually had doctors in the past tell us that they could make more money from other brokers that they've communicated with, but they've gone with us because of what we stood for, and for the culture that we create, knowing that their legacy will be not only protected but carried on.

The second half of the day, after that critical lunch period where you get face time together on an intimate level, is when you do need to go into your systems and what's in it for the doctors, the teams and the patients. It's critical to include what's in it for the teams and the patients, because this gives you the opportunity to put that question at ease. Two major questions we've seen with every doctor: 1) Are the patients being put first? 2) Is the team taken care of? One of the most important parts of the entire presentation is going to be related to the team and the patients. You want to make sure that the prospective doctor has the right information to answer the teams correctly when they return from this presentation. Otherwise, the deal could be ruined if the team were to throw up roadblocks, the context of his plan could be misunderstood, and ultimately, all of your efforts would have been in vain.

10

TRANSITIONING
THE NEW OFFICE

After purchasing our first five practices, we had developed some great relationships, one of which was with a practice broker who worked for one of the larger transition companies. This gentleman had actually sold four of our offices to us acting as our broker, so we had an established, trusting relationship. He actually still holds our record of quickest closing of an office, which was eleven days from beginning to end. Needless to say, our track record together provided a strong trust, but at the same time we didn't know what we didn't know. We didn't recognize how crucial due diligence and pre-closing action steps are to assure a successful transition, and also to protect yourself. You see, this gentleman brought us an office to purchase one day and it seemed like a goldmine deal. He presented the package as he always did, showed us the numbers, explained that we needed to move quickly and everything looked great, so we went all in.

Our lack of experience and recklessness came back to bite us hard. On day one, we were instantly in the hole with this office. For the year-and-a-half that we owned this office, we lost an average of $16,500 per month. We went with our gut, which was at the time based on the information we had, which was blind trust. We had no roadmap and knew no better. We didn't listen to our other advisers who said, "Slow down. Make sure you go through a solid due diligence process!," and we pulled the trigger. Little did we know that this broker illegally had ownership in the office, had misrepresented the office, and was trying to just unload it by taking advantage of our relationship.

Had we the robust due diligence checklist and systems that we now have in place, we would have uncovered the issues far before signing on the dotted line, and would not have the emotional scars that that office created. Our due diligence checklist and our pre-closing checklist were created over years of trial and error, to make sure the right people are looking at the right things. We're going to walk you through it step by step as an overview so that you don't make the same mistakes we made.

The first step is to do an in-depth financial review with your accountant. But there's a caveat to this: make sure your accountant is a dental-specific accountant and not a general accountant who does some dental accounting on the side. Make sure all tax-related documents, tax returns, P&L's, and a cash flow analysis for the previous three to five years are included. Make sure you set up a meeting between your accountant and the selling doctor's accountant. At some point they're going to be talking, no matter what, and will inevitably slow down the process unless they're introduced early on in the conversation. Two things slow down a transition: attorneys and accountants. We like to address it head-on and get the right parties talking sooner, knowing they're the ones who hold things up generally.

The second step is a walkthrough of the office. Schedule an office walkthrough either physically or with a video camera. In our experience, it's best if there are no team members there when you do this. Doctors are very cautious when discussing transition and acquisitions with their teams, and will generally protect their team from that conversation until it happens, or at least is getting closer to the dotted line. A lot of scarcity mentality is created inherently for team members, and it's not their fault. We've actually witnessed team members put a resignation letter in before the office even closes, out of fear of the transition and change. So being proactive with a doctor and letting them know that you support keeping it confidential is a must. Let them know that you can do a walkthrough on their terms, not yours. You'll develop better relationship capital and trust in the transition process. Here's one final thought on why it's critical to see the office. It may work for the existing doctor and the existing team, but what happens when you want to transition that doctor out and bring a new associate in? Is the office good for a prospective associate who wants to settle down in that area? Will you have to build a brand new building to make them happy, and invest a million dollars into a shell to have it be attractive to an associate? Remember, you're not necessarily buying this for yourself to practice in. You're buying this for other doctors to work in, with other needs and other desires, and you have to tailor it to that idea.

The third step is everything legal. After a Letter of Intent is signed, you have to begin the process of having your attorney customize closing documents to purchase the office, whether as an internal owner financing document or to submit to the bank. Furthermore, you need to have your attorney connect with the selling doctor's attorney early on, because attorneys will generally slow down the process, even more than accountants. We've never met an attorney yet who wants to make the process easy and just roll over and agree with the contract terms that you want as the purchaser. You can expect several exchanges back and forth and this is where emotions can run high. It's best to let the attorneys do their work and be the mediators of this process; You do not want to be caught in the middle while emotions are high negotiating contract terms, as it can put pebbles in the shoe of the relationship and damage the momentum that you have with a future selling doctor. We actually walked away from a deal in 2015 with a practice because during contract negotiations, the doctor proved to be extremely difficult to work with and not true partner material.

The fourth step is an on-site equipment analysis and fee schedule report. This is vital because you could take over an office and two months later have a compressor go down, costing you $8,000 to $12,000 right off the bat. You need a forecast of the equipment that may need to be replaced before moving forward. Furthermore, getting a fee schedule analysis is an important step in analyzing the office. For our organization, this has been driven by a program one of the big three supply companies provides in which they'll do an analysis of lost income potential. It's just another piece of the potential puzzle that allows you to see whether there's opportunity in the office or lack of opportunity. If that doctor is at the 90th percentile for fee schedule in the surrounding ten mile radius, there's not a lot of room to play with the fees. However, if they're at the 30th percentile for all procedures, you know that you have an opportunity to create an appropriate game plan be able to raise the fees and have instant profitability for that practice. On a related note, if that doctor is only at the 50th percentile but your plan is to raise them to the 70th or 90th percentile, you're going to have to discuss this with the doctor that you're going to keep on prior to closing. It's possible he/she won't agree to it. We had an office that was established in a small community for 35 years, and the doctor was really worried about earning a bad reputation for the office if we changed anything with the fee schedule. They don't think that they deserve prices that are in the 90th percentile, or that their office isn't nice enough to be able to offer prices in the 90th percentile. Therefore, they won't stand behind the treatment plans. Nobody wins in that scenario.

The fifth step is to hire an I.T. company to do a full computer hardware and software analysis. We treat this as a separate, additional step to auditing their overall equipment status because in our experience, it is usually this area that needs the most immediate attention. For some reason, in all the offices we've looked at and transitioned, the doctors seemed to have the mentality that the computers are the last to update and if it's working well enough, that's just fine and dandy. However, as it relates to HIPAA guidelines, there are upgrades to the software operating systems that have to be done, and you're out of compliance if you don't make the upgrades; many, many offices are out of compliance in our experience. Just to remain HIPAA-compliant with the most up-to-date operating system generally requires a rather beefy server and rather beefy satellite computers. Unfortunately, that usually requires a revamp of the entire network. It will cost at least $20,000 to $25,000 for an average office to get new computers, a new server and an upgraded operating system. As you become bigger, you'll have a larger target on your back, and will get to the point that you have no choice but to make these investments to remain HIPAA compliant and OSHA compliant in every office.

The sixth step is to have a pre-closing business office setup checklist, that is quarterbacked by one individual on your team, to make sure the proper bank accounts are set up. Banks generally require four weeks or more prior to closing to have accounts properly set up to have check scanners ordered and have time to set up before the close.

Finally, you're going to set a closing date and be prepared to sign all the documents on that closing date. Our initial protocol was to always print four physical copies, fly to the location, have a celebratory event and all sign together. This methodology does create a great context of a new future together and it worked for many years. We strongly advocate using DocuSign as an account for your signatures because it creates a searchable, complete digital document on day one of your contracts that you'll always have easy access to. There will be times when you need to reference them, and if you had hard copies that were later scanned, there's a chance for error and the chance for missing a page.

So what happens on closing day? We have two very special protocols that we have mastered in creating a great relationship at the point of transition. It is your responsibility to start creating the context of the year ahead. We do it by means of an on-site, one day kick-off seminar for the entire team.

The most important aspect of our on-site kick-off seminar is that we create an emotional event for the doctor and the team in the form of a team workshop. This seminar is the first step in developing a trusting relationship with the team, and it begins with great rapport. This is an intense, full-day team workshop at the office to get everyone engaged and connected. It's an outcome-based seminar, so the very first thing we go over with the team is what the outcomes of the day will be. This is where you start creating the context of the year ahead. This is where you start getting them excited to follow your lead. This is where you show them what your vision is, what your mission is.

There are two major exercises that we quarterback that day for the team. In both of these exercises, we are merely the facilitator; the majority of the work is done by the team. The first one is called The Life Story Exercise. This is a mind-blowing exercise for the team members in which they start to develop relationships with each other on a deeper level. It never fails when we do this exercise, there are tears, hugs and breakthroughs by the end of the exercise!

We believe in the tell-show-do methodology, so we do The Life Story Exercise personally first to show them the format. This is your huge opportunity for the team to get to know their new leader! We make sure we go into great detail, that we get into our personal lives, our families, etc. The exercise is then for each team member to write down their life story for ten minutes. We get everyone around in a circle and every team member reads their life story out loud. The final part of the exercise is to give everyone the opportunity to acknowledge their fellow team member. For the selling doctor, this is an incredible opportunity to give acknowledgments and appreciation for your team members. The point of this exercise is not to expose everyone's vulnerabilities; it's optional and people only discuss what they choose. What it does is to allow everyone to recognize what they've learned from the past, put the past in the past, acknowledge that it's in the past and needs to stay there, and draw a line in the sand, step over and create a new future with a blank slate starting that day. It's an emotional cleanse. People will carry the past on their shoulders and let it affect their present and future if they don't step back and recognize it.

The next part of this one-day kick-off seminar is an overview of your organization. You're going to tell your story and the history of it. You're going to explain your management protocols. You're going to give them certainty in this transition and in your leadership. You're going to show your strength and experience. When we do our overview, we make sure we include our eight divisions of management and what role each of those division directors encompasses.

The second half of the day is what we call the Mission, Vision, Core Value Statement Exercise. It is absolutely critical that you share with the team exactly what your mission, vision, and value statement is for your organization, but that it is likely not theirs. Because you can't force your vision, purpose and values on an office, and we recognized this early on, we created a hands-on exercise that allows the team to feel empowered, and united, and create their own mission, vision and core values. In this exercise, you act as the mediator and guide them on a pathway towards creating a blank slate for the office, in which they take ownership of the future of the office, where they feel empowered and as a team create a vision they can stand behind.

We always see awesome mission statements posted on dentists' websites, and over time they all blend in and seem generic; you can almost tell a marketing company suggested them for the doctor. But did the team have any real input in that? What we found in the past was that they usually were shown a quick statement by the doctor before it was posted on the website company and asked, "Do you like this?" And up it goes. Is it any surprise that the team is not united behind the mission and vision of the office? The success of our group management model depends greatly on the entire team as a whole, uniting them with a great purpose is paramount.

If you want to reset the context for the entire future of the team and onboard them as empowered individuals, they have to be part of the big, juicy future of this office, and feel like they own the future. So in this exercise, we have everybody take a pad of paper and a pen and sit in a circle. We have a big whiteboard behind us, or a projector, to take notes so everyone can see the progress of the exercise. We begin by asking a series of questions. The first question we ask relates to the mission, which is the "why" or the reason the office exists. And then we follow by asking them five questions. One, why are they in the practice of dentistry; Two, how would they like their patients to view them; Three, what level of service do they wish to provide for their patients; Four, outside of bread and butter dentistry, what else would they like your practice to be known for; Five, how are they different from other practices in the area? We give everyone two minutes to write down one-to three-word, short phrases of all the ideas that pop into their heads that are in-line with their own values and perceptions of the office.

After everybody answers each question for two minutes, we have everybody share their answers out loud, and we write them all down on a whiteboard where everybody can see. We do this for every question under "mission" and end up with a pretty long list of one-to three-word phrases that represent the collective knowledge and the collective ideas of every single team member engaged in full-on participation. The final step is to create a voting system to guide them in narrowing all of those phrases down to one sentence that describes the mission of the office (See Diagram 15). You get a lot of back and forth and a lot of excitement and debate. We've never had an office that then doesn't come up with a final mission phrase that they all feel united behind. It's a powerful team workshop exercise that's all about inclusion. Clearly it's much different than a marketing company making a suggestion for you or really just something the doctor created.

We then do the exact same thing for the vision or the "where" the office is going. We ask four questions: One, what will the practice look like in five years; Two, how will the community perceive the practice in five years; Three, how will the dental community view the practice in five years; Four, how will the team remain true to their roots as they grow? And again, after all team members collectively have had their input, we narrow it down to one vision statement.

Finally, we do the same thing for core values, but it's only one question per team member and that is: What are your three core values? And we come up with three core values as a team that everyone is united behind. We have an incredible mission, vision, core value statement that is generally done within the first week of transition and sets the context for that big, juicy future.

The final step is to memorialize it. For under $300, you can have the big chain print companies take this phrase and put it into a graphic that is a banner stand (see Diagram 16). We found that having two, one in the waiting room and one in the break room, is a fresh, six-foot tall reminder of the mission, vision, core values that the office stands for. It's just a nice little physical touch to memorialize a concept, and it's inexpensive and easy to do.

Infinity Dental offers a solution for a dentist no matter what stage of their career cycle they are in. We actually developed a protocol called Developing your Life Plan that shows how you can grow through a series of phases within our organization, based on your personal vision and what endpoint you choose. One unique solution we offer is a 50-50 partnership plan, in which our original partnership (between the two of us) is modeled into a successful growth model with which other dentists can participate. When we do a 50-50 partnership transition, we have an additional key protocol to start the partnership off in the right context, and empower us through great communication towards a big future.

Partnerships can be tricky because they necessitate a shared decision-making process, and if you're reading this book, you are likely going to be the silent non-practicing partner in the equation. So the position you're coming from is one of trust and reliance based on the feedback from the practicing partner. We created an exercise called a Partnership Alignment Profile Exercise that we do the evening of the one-day seminar to keep the momentum of that exciting day going, and to start the partnership off right. This partnership profile is doctor-to-doctor and is done in a private setting, generally during or after dinner. It's critical to know the personality profile of your partners so you know what works and what doesn't in communication.

The first aspect we review is our core values individually, and we see where they are aligned or misaligned. This is where each partner writes down their core values, even though it was already discussed in the one-day exercise earlier in the day. This is partner-to-partner and sometimes there are things that come out that a doctor won't say in front of their team. This allows you to get to the heart of what makes that doctor tick, and allows them to see your core values. It allows you to see where there's alignment in values and also where there may not be, which gives you insight in conflict management.

The next things we review are our strengths and weaknesses. This is a time when vulnerability is an asset and you can comfortably open up, because it's the vulnerabilities that you have, that you're willing to express, that creates transparency. This allows your partner to respect those vulnerabilities, and if they are great partner, make up for them. It also shows your strengths that may compliment your partner's weaknesses. By the end of this exercise, you'll start seeing where you're aligned, where you're not, and how you can compliment each other in a successful business strategy of great communication.

Next, we go over our Rules. These are our must-haves. These are boundaries that are not crossed, agreements of how we operate and how we move forward.

Finally, we set one-year and three-year goals. We need to know where the partnership is headed so we can reverse-engineer a strategy in the short term and the longer term, to make sure all partners are happy.

11

PRACTICE MANAGEMENT AND TEAM TRAINING

Practice management and team training go hand-in-hand. If you train your teams properly to operate by specific systems, and you create a culture of empowerment, they inherently manage themselves and the practice runs smoothly. It's the paradigm shift from saying, "I'll hire a manager to manage the team and the office" to "I'll train my team intensely with systems to manage themselves." Empowered, well-trained individuals united toward a common goal outperform micro-managed mice every day of the week. Here's the problem with the current model of management and training: it's expensive, it requires on-site personnel or expensive off-site trips, it's disempowering, it's not scalable, it's not easily duplicatable, it can be inconsistent, and the list goes on and on. Here's what we do know team members and doctors love, and which is very effective: team workshops.

Over the last eight years we have spent over $1.2 million dollars cash on consulting, training, and seminars to learn how to best manage and train our employees. Getting that knowledge and experience to all of our teams has been difficult at best. That's why we created the world's first digital comprehensive dental training program, Infinity Dental University, to transform employees from working independently, and focusing on their own little area, to working together as a highly functional TEAM that creates a WOW experience for the patient. The program is centered around a series of two-week, on-site team workshops that conveniently take place in the practice. No more costly consulting trips, no more shutting the office down, no more spreading the cost out over years. It's hardcore, boot-camp style training every two weeks!

We spent eight years perfecting this powerful dental practice training program that encompassed the following three goals: 1) improve the patient's experience when they come to your office, 2) make every employee's job easier to perform, and 3) increase collections within the first year of implementation. We have an advantage over most dentists. We have been applying and testing these strategies in our offices as we practiced. Recognizing this fact, our University comes with a highly trained personal coach who oversees its implementation in the first year. Having someone dedicated to the office, coaching and overseeing the implementation of the training provided in the University really enhances the probability of success and achieving a major breakthrough in the offices. As a result, we developed a system for training dental team members that works like crazy.

We had a rule within our University. Our rule was to commit to real on-the-job training of everything we ever learned, and test every system on our own practices to make sure these strategies worked. If they didn't hold up and meet one of the three criteria, 1) improve the patient experience, 2) make an employee's job easier, or 3) increase the profitability of the practice, then we didn't include it in our University and bring it to the rest of the offices.

We created our Four Pillars Of Training Dental Employees. We're going to list these four really quickly and then we're going to go through each one in more detail.

1. Research and test
2. Turn into an online video training module
3. Coach on its implementation into your practice
4. Testing and accountability

Pillar One – Research and Test. We know that there is always more to learn about effectively training employees to work as highly functional team members. So we are always looking for nuggets of wisdom that other people have found which can be applied to our dental practices. Once we find what appears to be a good fit, we then must test it to validate that it will work in any dental office, regardless of the DNA makeup of that office.

Pillar Two – Turn it Into an Online Training Module. Once we have tested and validated that a new training system will work, we then have to turn it into a video. That video is then uploaded online so that it is available 24/7. We turn it into an online video because that is how people learn in today's digital environment. We also want them to have access to the video 24/7 so that they can review it at any time, day or night. The problem with other training systems is that they are dependent on the availability of either the doctor or the office manager, which makes it awkward to train an employee.

Pillar Three – Coach on Its Implementation Into Your Practice. If you are like us, you hired consultants who said they could help you. But what we found was that they expected the doctor to implement their recommendations. And although we wanted to take advantage of the recommendations, we were too busy running the office and treating patients to take on the extra responsibility of training the staff in new methods that we weren't one-hundred percent positive would work.

We realized when we created Infinity Dental University that we had to have a coach who could oversee its implementation, and coach employees on how the new system or tactic would affect their jobs. So, our University comes with a well-trained coach to implement the modules into your practice. That doesn't mean that the doctors aren't involved, but the time they spend on working with your coach is a small fraction compared to what they would spend if they were to oversee the implementation on their own.

Pillar Four – Testing and Accountability. It is our experience that an employee will just blow things off unless they are held accountable to somebody. As a result, we will test the employees after every module to make sure that they reviewed the module and understand what they are learning. We hold a brief meeting weekly with your team and they are accountable to our coach, and have the opportunity to ask questions if they didn't understand something.

Because our management program and philosophy is so centered around great training, we want to include details on what just one year of our four-year program looks like. After you go through it, we hope you'll see how the program as a whole creates an office that is both well-trained and well-managed.

Two-week Pre-Launch Videos

Context vs. Content: Team members will learn how we set up the University videos into two elements: The "Content" of the module, or "why" that module is important from a provider's perspective is explained, then contrasted with the "Content" of the video, or "how" these robust modules are implemented into the office.

Integrity: Team members learn how the Education Facilitator operates with integrity, in terms of scheduling and showing up for coaching sessions, following through with their implementation, and playing all-out the entire time when the in-house University workshops are being delivered.

Roles and Responsibilities: Each team member will explain and document their specific roles and responsibilities within the office so the implementation of the University can be centered around the right people in the right places.

Module #1: Mission, Vision, Value Statement Creation

The problem with most missions/visions is that they are created by the doctor or a marketing team; very rarely do they include the input of the entire team. Start the year out strong with developing a united mission and vision created from the collective inputs of every team member in a hands-on workshop that allows the office to "blank slate" their future and unite as a team. After a mission, vision, value statement is created, team members learn how to use it in their office every day and how to display it with pride to their patients. Values: Team unification, direction for the office, purpose-driven teams.

Module #2: Interpersonal Communication System For The Team

Communication is everything. To start IDU's one year program, we set up the doctor and the team with the concept of managing by agreements. We know that all upsets in life are a result of either a missing agreement or a broken agreement. In this module, we teach how to identify the missing agreements in the office as a team, and then write them down in a monthly log book that the office reviews on a regular basis. Furthermore, we teach conflict resolution and how to effectively tackle any issue between team members systematically, and integrate them into the agreement book. Finally, we teach how to manage difficult team members who continue to lack integrity and break their existing agreements by using the AIDE system - Ask, Insist, Demand, Enforce. Value: Greatly reduced stress, better team unity, better organization to the office.

Module #3: Team Bonus System

The team is finally going to have a system that acknowledges them for their hard work. We developed a monthly team bonus system to incentivize every position within the office based on their performance. First, we calculate the lost income potential of the office based on their existing active patient base, and show what's currently possible within their office. Next, we calculate a responsible monthly goal, and individual goals per position, based on production and tasks that increase profitability. Finally, we calculate the monthly overhead of the office, make sure the office puts away enough for retirement, growth, rainy days, bonus payment, and vacations, and then reverse engineer our proven module that links bonuses to case acceptance for every department. We teach the team how to track their progress and work together toward progressively increasing the overall monthly production and collections of the office. We integrate a tracking system that allows one team member to quarterback and report to everyone.

Value: Explosive team-driven growth, team empowerment, increased case acceptance.

Module #4: Hygiene Incentive Program

Dental hygienists are the second highest producers in the office, and account for 20-30% of the total office production. They are also the main touchpoint for patient education. Our incentive program for dental hygienists allows them to get commissioned on selling auxiliary products and procedures that increase the office production. The incentive program is taught as an additional bonus on top of their existing wage to create a lucrative opportunity for hygienists to not only sustain their existing financial certainty, but make more when they educate patients more. Value: Increased practice production, healthier patients, happier hygienists.

Module #5: Creating Uniform Treatment Plans

Many offices struggle with reading the doctor's mind in terms of diagnosis and treatment planning clinically. When everyone is on the same page, it creates certainty for patients and team members, and allows the team to unite toward one message. This module creates uniformity between multiple providers, both hygienists and doctors, for scheduling and treatment planning purposes, by creating a structured checklist on every procedure in the office. Implemented as a workshop-style module, it allows collaboration and documentation for existing and future team members.   Value: Confidence amongst team members, a clear message to patients, easier expansion with new providers.

Module #6: Checklists To Run The Office

Create sustained structure by a series of checklist systems that allow you to hire based on personality and attitude, not off of skill. The ultimate accountability is created for every team member by a series of daily, weekly, monthly and annual checklists that can be audited.   Team members customize their own checklists in this module that integrates the unique attributes of their office, yet follows a proven standard for success.   Team members now have the ability to self-manage their positions and doctors can have the confidence that every aspect of the office is run like a machine.   Value: Structure to manage every position, accountability for team members.

Module #7: Software That Measures The Daily Health Of The Office

We co-created a robust practice management software that measures the daily, weekly and monthly most critical numbers, per position, of the office. It is the first dental software of its kind that takes measurements of daily performance from a numbers perspective and can translate the information into the clinical health of the office. Doctors are able to see what areas are weak and require extra attention. Utilizing daily goals and email alerts, team members have a system to measure themselves against national standards of a healthy office. With less than 5 minutes of input from each team member at the end of each day, doctors will be able to measure and see each aspect of the office through the lens of a CFO. Value: Immediate measurement of weak areas of office, a dashboard report of the office numbers that matter, increased accountability.

Module #8: A Structured Morning Meeting

Implement a time-tested specific structure for a morning meeting that will increase communication and be outcome-oriented from every department. Our morning meetings focus on three things: 1). Opportunities for same day dentistry, 2). Opportunities to re-engage old treatment plans in hygiene, 3). Opportunities to engage in rapport development with patients. There are alway patients who slip through the cracks in every office, and this system gets the team united toward putting a cork in it. Also, when the team is united towards connecting with patients at a deeper level of the patient experience, it creates trust amongst patients and a high internal referral rate. Value: Getting everyone on the same page every day, a structured meeting that gets to what actually matters, and a way to account for every treatment plan coming through hygiene.

Module #9: Standardizing Care For The Team

It's one thing for providers to get on the same page with treatment planning, but the real power comes when the entire team can communicate *to patients* what the office stands for, why the patient needs to be at a better level of health, and how to get them there. We create a visual aid that can be used in handouts, on the wall, or on a computer screen for patients. It presents a united front on the standard of care the office stands for in the community. Then, we teach how to communicate this powerful tool in the patient workflow with the intention of unprecedented patient communication, leading to increased case acceptance. Value: Team unification in the mission of the office, better patient education, increased case acceptance.

Module #10: Matching Treatment To A Patient's Lifestyle
Patients often put off dentistry because they don't value it enough in their life. This module teaches team members how to educate patients on their specific conditions and how to link it to the most important things in their life. Teams will learn how to make dentistry a want, not a need, in the patient's mind. We provide specific strategies to dig for patient's lifestyle indicators utilizing 3 specific method-ologies. We also show how even with minimal success, team members have a new strategy to listen "for" when patients speak, not "to," and therefore connect at a deeper level. Value: Improved patient experience, better communication on the importance of dentistry, higher case acceptance.

Module #11: Creating A Sense Of Urgency For Treatment

Too often providers go straight from diagnosing problems to providing solutions. Unfortunately, they forget the most important element: Consequences. Consequences are "why" the patient should care about the treatment being suggested. We teach how to put scarcity mentality into a patient by teaching how to effectively communicate the consequences of delaying treatment. In conjugation with lifestyle indicators and educating on a standard of care, discussing consequences of inaction helps increase case acceptance. The team will unite behind creating a sense of urgency and utilize it as a motivational tool for patients. Value: Increased case acceptance.

Module #12: Streamlining Exams With The Hygiene Hand-Off Form

Create the perfect transfer of information between hygienist and doctor with this simple form that will greatly increase the effectiveness of the patient exam, and also learn when to implement it during the hygiene patient appointment. The form has all the demographic information that actually matters for rapport development for the doctor, and includes all of the important clinical findings in the hygiene evaluation to help guarantee nothing is missed in the treatment plan. Value: Decreased stress for the doctor at exams, increased production.

Module #13: Creating The Treatment Coordinator Position
Utilizing a Treatment Coordinator position with defined roles and responsibilities is a critical step in the workflow of the patient experience. We teach how to create the position, and what the protocols and scripts are. We provide patient education tools to have at their disposal, and teach them how to effectively close the deal. Patients love having a separate space with a separate advocate to help find a way to fit treatment into their busy lives   and their financial situations.   Value: Increased case acceptance, guaranteed lower accounts receivables, structure in the patient process.

Module #14: Payment Arrangements That Increase Case Acceptance
We teach a protocol that is a simple breakdown of the treatment plan and treatment payment options that becomes a powerful tool for a treatment coordinator to use with every patient in the workflow process. Patients are provided with three convenient options, including an in-house short term payment plan, to provide flexibility in getting their treatment completed. We use a specific form that patients can bring home that explains their treatment plan and what plan they selected for payment. Value: Payment options for patients, better communication about finances, increased case acceptance, better cash flow.

Module #15: The Ideal Patient Workflow

Learn as a team to master the patient experience from the moment the patient walks in the door to when they leave, with time-tested techniques that provide a world-class, predictable workflow. Furthermore, learn how to transfer treatment plan information between each team member to create clarity and enrollment of patients. There's a right way and a wrong way to take a patient through the process. The method you use can lead to either increased case acceptance or delay of treatment for another six months. This workflow process creates a predictable assembly line of hand-offs between providers to ensure value is created in a systematic way. Value: Increase case acceptance, better communication to patients, better patient experience, increased referrals.

Module #16: Controlling The Patient Experience With Checklists

Why leave the world-class patient experience just created to chance? We create a checklist system that follows every patient. This guarantees uniformity for every patient and truly brand the practice around the experience. The team learns who is responsible for what in the checklist, how it follows the patient and how to hand it off properly to other team members. The team will have a specific form to use as an example, but will be coached on how to customize it to the genetics of their own office. Value: Consistency in the patient experience, increased referrals.

Module #17: Scheduling That Maximizes Productivity

Learn how to finally connect both the scheduling team in the front and the clinical team in the back with a system that fosters unprecedented communication, creating schedules that flow smoothly. The team will learn how to do a time study that is customized to every doctor in their office, and gives an accurate account of how the doctor currently practices. Then, that information is put into a communication system that enables you to schedule providers to maximize their production potential. Value: Smoother schedules, no gaps in the schedule, a harmonious front and back, maximized productivity every day, patients who are seated on time.

Module #18: Splitting The Schedule Into Easier Workloads

The traditional way for doctors to practice fills their days with an equal mix of hygiene exams and a productive schedule in their chair of clinical dentistry. That balance can create undue stress when there is a better way! The team will learn how to schedule the doctor into exam-heavy days and operative-heavy days to create less stress, better clinical care, and an actual guaranteed bump in production. Value: Less stress for doctors, better focus on their clinical care, happier hygienists.

Module #19: Phone Scripts That Make A Predictable 1st Impression

The front desk associates learn what to say and what not to say for the 21st-century patient. They will learn why it's crucial not to ask for insurance over the phone and learn key tips on how to create a great first impression. Specific scripts are discussed and implemented to give certainty in the conversation, and avoid pitfalls that consume time and don't get the patient in the door. Value: Increased conversion of new patients from phone, less time wasted tied up on the phones, more productive schedule.

Module #20: Soft Tissue Management Program

Hygienists will learn a time-tested, step-by-step protocol to educate patients on the intricacies and options involved in keeping their gums healthy long term. Periodontal disease can be difficult for patients to understand, difficult to articulate for case acceptance, and is often under-diagnosed. This program acts a roadmap to a healthy mouth with every patient, so no one slips through the cracks. The team will learn terminology that makes sense to patients and tips and tricks of our proven soft tissue management program. Value: Increased periodontal disease diagnosis, increased office production, healthier patients, decreased liability as an office.

Module #21: Auxiliary Chairside Services

In this module you're going to learn implementation protocols for several critical services for your patients, and learn how to implement these money-making tools with all patients. We go into detail on oral cDNA, sealants, flouride, in-house whitening, and whitening tray impressions and how to get your team to drive their integration into the patient experience. Value: Increased production, healthier patients.

Module #22: Digital Diagnostic Tools That Increase Case Acceptance

This module teaches the clinical team tips, tricks and ideal implementation, from a provider's perspective, on three crucial diagnostic devices, and how to use the information in front of a patient to get them onboard with their treatment. Spectra, Diagnodent and Intra-oral cameras are covered extensively so that the clinical team has a foundation to make an agreement for use with every single patient. Value: Increased case acceptance, increased patient education.

Module #23: Implementing An Extended Warranty System

Never worry about a redo on-the-house and give patients massive value by including this service and knowing how to script it. Give patients peace of mind with an extended warranty, and you are guaranteed full fee reimbursement for any redone work. Value: No more give-aways, patient peace of mind with their treatment.

Module #24: An Audit System to Protect The Practice

Learn how to guarantee lasting implementation of all of the office improvements by a methodology to spread accountability and delegate simple audits for long-term implementation. Doctors and team leaders will have a protocol utilizing a specific form to keep a healthy eye on the practice. Value: Certainty that all of the processes implemented last, sustained practice infrastructure.

Module #25: Branding And Marketing

Nowadays, everything is branding! Brand, brand, brand!! This module is going to teach the team how to uniquely brand the office in a way that will provide a competitive edge in the community. The team will also learn how to market the new unique brand. Value: Branded practice, increased marketing potential, more new patients.

Module #26: Internal Referral System The Team Can Run

Everyone knows internal marketing is the most effective way to new patients, and at this point in the University, the team has laid the foundation for an unbelievable patient experience. This module will teach how to convert that experience to a steady supply of new patients in an effective internal referral system. Value: Increased new patient count, decreased marketing overhead.

Module #27. Bringing It All Together By Creating Team Manuals

Every position, with every role, responsibility, checklist and process, has been optimized sequentially and now must be documented and made duplicatable. As the practice grows, new team members must be brought up to speed quickly. In this module, we enroll the team members to systematically create a training manual for their position over the course of one month to guarantee longevity to their improvements. Value: Longevity to the practice improvements, stability when change happens.

12

FINDING AND
ONBOARDING
ASSOCIATES

Over the years, we have found that one of the most important aspects of running a group practice is managing your doctors. Again, they account for 70% to 80% of the collections coming into your organization, so they deserve 70% to 80% of your attention. Team members come and go. Doctors are less transient over the years. That also comes with some major challenges. Doctor can have egos. Doctor are usually highly motivated. Doctors have different wants and needs than team members. And great doctors can be harder to find. It's becoming an increasingly competitive environment to find associates because small groups and solo practitioners are competing with large groups. Large DSO's get to them far faster because they have more resources, and quite honestly at times are more attractive to an associate fresh out of school.

Let's talk about the ideal associate. The ideal associate has been out practicing for three years. An associate fresh out of school is not up to speed yet clinically, and will require six to twelve months of transition just to get their speed up. Also, they have not had time to get into any higher level clinical procedures, such as placing implants or Invisalign, because in those first years they're really just focusing on gaining speed and getting comfortable.

On the flip side of that coin, after much more than three years of experience, they are hard to mold. A doctor who's been working for ten to fifteen years has become set in his ways. It can be difficult to get them to adapt to a different philosophy and get them on board with the culture of your group.

At three years, they are up to speed, and have learned some higher level procedures, yet are still moldable to the culture of your group. Now, you might think that the ideal associate is one just like you: one who's motivated, experienced, driven, happy, excited, inspirational, and who every patient loves. You may be shocked to know that none of that stuff really matters much. The reality is that the ideal associate is one who is a great producer and who is free of drama, and who doesn't create problems in the office.

Let us explain, and this comes from a lot of experience and frustrations. Somebody who's just like you, who's incredibly driven, isn't going to stick around very long, and will be driven to start their own practice or leave your group after getting what they wanted out of you. We've had so many associates over the years. What we found is that as long as they consistently produce on a monthly basis and are not creating problems in the office with the team and the patients, they are the Steady Eddys that keeps the office moving forward. We know that's counter-intuitive to what you think and it's not even natural to think that way, but this is experience talking, and this is where you have to rely on others in the industry who have gone down this route.

There is a plethora of ways to find associates, and we've tried them all (or at least it feels that way). Sometimes it's a matter of hustling and literally going to schools, putting posts on every website possible, putting ads in every journal, etc. But there is a more efficient way and that is Placement Programs. As an organization, we have invested in five placement programs. These came with an initial investment of $9,000 to $15,000 just to get on their program, but they have opened up many doors for us. In a nutshell, an associate placement program is a company that gives you access to their list of available candidates. They work with you intimately to talk about your individual practice or practices, what you're searching for, and what you would consider your ideal candidate. Then when the time comes that you need a new associate, they put the word out and make the connection between you and the prospective doctor. They do a trust transfer at that point to edify your group and you as the CEO to set up the relationship properly. After that, it's up you to bring them into your office and on board them properly.

The investment for an associate through a placement programs averages between $8,000 and $9,000. However, you generally have 90 days before you have to pay. Furthermore, if that associate does not work out in the first 90 days, you don't have to pay anything. So you're closer to a guarantee of having somebody who's going to work out in the office.

Now let's talk about onboarding your associates. This is a critical process to a successful transition. Associates are looking for certainty right off the bat, and a future with your office. Providing certainty is number one. They've got big debts, big bills, and generally a family to feed. So you have to be that rock that they can rely on, and they need to know that you were the right choice amongst all the options out there. Every moment you spend in the beginning onboarding an associate creates trust, and will pay out in dividends of starting a great relationship.

We've created what we call our Associate Onboarding Checklist. It's a series of interactions with the team, with patients, and with the associate to make sure that no stone is left unturned in terms of expectations, and it helps guarantee a successful transition. When you're talking about someone who's going to produce $800,000 for your organization every year, you don't want to leave anything to chance, and you want to make sure they start off right.

The first area that you have to work on is onboarding the team, and getting the team set up with the right expectations and knowledge of how to handle a new associate properly. Start with the obvious: Schedule a time to sit down and let the team know you're going to be bringing a new associate into the office. At this meeting you are going to discuss the associate's start date, what the expectations are with the associate, and what might come up in the process. Next, you'll discuss the schedule. You have to discuss and make an agreement on how new patients will be integrated between multiple doctors and how that's going to be broken up. How will you schedule the new doctor versus the existing doctors? Finally, you have to edify and champion the new associate to the team so they get excited about the transition. Make sure you identify "what's in it for them."

As a group practice owner, this is something you need to be sensitive to; that is, making sure your team creates a positive environment on day one, and is championing the associate to all of the new patients and all of the existing patients. The worst thing that can happen is for the team to display a lack of enthusiasm for their new doc. The final aspect you're going to do, as it relates to onboarding the associate with your team, is to have the associate come in and meet the team. You really want all the team members to interact with the associate, and it's crucial for you or your management team to champion each team member to the associate. The associate needs to see that it's a unified team. Again, your role here is going to be championing and edifying the doctor to the team, and also championing and edifying the team to the doctor. This is critical to promote great culture and to start it off right. Remember, culture is everything.

Next, you're going to have the associate come in and visit the practice while it's running. It's important for them to see the daily dynamics, as every office is different. They need to understand how each team member works in every department. We actually recommend having the associate sit down with each team member for 20 to 30 minutes and learn what they do and how they do it. This provides individual time with each team member to develop a strong working relationship with the associate, but also allows the associate to have empathy towards the team members in their positions and understand how the practice works.

The associate needs to understand the details of the practice. They need to know about any agreements in the office, roles and responsibilities of each team member, the mission, vision, and core values of the practice, and the office manual. One of your management team members needs to go through your office manual for that practice so there is a solid understanding of your expectations. Your assistants, or whoever is responsible for ordering the dental supplies, need to walk the associate to the inventory and go over all the items that are used in the office, and how they are used. There may be some dental materials they are not used to, so it's critical to go over that prior to having the first patient in the chair!

One of the biggest issues we've seen over the years is that associates love to come in and just start ordering all new stuff! They will drive a bill through the roof on ordering very quickly if you give them free rein to do this. Do not do this! Associates can come and go and we've made it a policy in our group that there are no new materials being ordered in the first 90 days, unless they go through a very specific process and they've had to work for it to prove why this new product is necessary. We've had it happen on several occasions where we've dropped $8,000 to $12,000 on new supplies and equipment for an associate, who didn't work out 60 days later, and that stuff just got shelved because no one else used it. You want an associate who can adapt their techniques to your materials from your proven list, that you know work well. If they can't adapt, they're not great associates, or at least it's a check against them.

The senior dentist and the assistant need to sit down with the associate prior to seeing patients and become familiar with the operatory. They need to go over all the existing dental equipment, the handpieces, how the chair works, how the curing lights work, how the practice management software works, etc., so that on day one when they hit the ground running seeing patients, there are no awkward conversations that lose trust with the patient. Nothing loses trust faster than fumbling with the chair or not knowing how a handpiece works. It's absolutely critical that this has been walked through several times prior to seeing the first patient.

The next big area that you have to work on with transitioning an associate is the patients. It obviously starts with the first point of contact: Scheduling. Your front desk associate should notify operative patients in the dentist's schedule, not hygiene patients, at the time of confirming the appointments, that the associate will be seeing them. Hygiene patients can be scheduled normally and can be made aware once they are in their appointment. It's a very big mistake to just surprise a patient and have a new doctor show up to actually do the dentistry. No one likes those kinds of surprises, especially when they've been expecting to see the same doctor they've know for a long time.

You're going to have some patients who will insist that they don't want to see another doctor, but in our experience the majority of the time it's not an issue. It all comes down to how you champion the new associate, and how you edify them to your patients. Here's a wonderful way to help with that process: When any existing patient goes to the new associate, ideally the senior dentist should personally introduce the associate to the patients and do a trust transfer. This can be literally as quick as stopping in the room for 15 seconds and introducing them and throwing in a quick one-liner of how they're going to love the new doctor! This does not take any longer than that, but is a critical part of transitioning the patient from old doctor to new doctor.

When I (Jared) first started practicing in my two offices, Dr. Charles Keever would come in with every patient and just say, "Hey Mr. Doe, you're going to love Dr. Van Ittersum. He's been with us now for the last couple of months and does fantastic work and everyone loves him. I know you're going to have a great experience. Have a great day." That's all it takes. When Dr. Achey would stop in to champion me to a new patient, he would say, "I'm so excited for you to work with my new partner, Dr. Van Ittersum. You guys are going to have a great experience." Again, it doesn't require more than that.

The other critical aspect of transferring patients to your new doctor is having your team unite behind the new associate in front of the patient. Whether it's a hygienist or the front desk, they always need to be edifying and championing the associate to the patient. The new associate needs to write up a solid one-page autobiography explaining what they do personally in their lives, so that connection can be made with patients. They need to make a list of some of the unique procedures they do in dentistry so team members can discuss that with patients. Your team needs to know what these aspects are and study this information so that when a patient that comes in that say, loves to fish, and the associate loves to fish, the team member could instantly make that connection and get the patient excited to see the associate to talk about fishing.

Your front desk associates needs to go over scheduling of patients with the associate doctor. The doctor needs to see how the schedule works so they can work the time flow in their mind. We all know as practicing doctors that you've got a time clock in your head and you know where you are with your patient, in terms of when your next patient is going to be coming in, and how that patient flow occurs. It's important that they understand how the schedule works in the office, so they can visualize the day ahead of time, and know exactly how much time there is, and they can also communicate how much time they need on the schedule for certain procedures. The worst thing you can do is have the timing off on the first several weeks with patients. As the senior doc, you may be able to do a crown prep in an hour with your eyes closed, but they may need an hour and 15 minutes. Having this communicated prior to scheduling is critical so that it's a smooth experience with your patients.

One way to set up the scheduling is by doing the ideal day exercise. Ask the critical question, "What is your ideal day? What does that look like to you? How many rooms are you using?" The reason that this is important is that you want to make sure that their ideal day works well with the way the office is currently set up. You may utilize block scheduling. You may have days where only exams are done. You want to make sure that you fit well within their dream schedule. If not, you need to talk about this before they start working on their first day.

We use several labs that give us group discounts, so we make sure there's an emphasis on those labs and that the associate ideally uses them. It's another great aspect of our associate placement program, that by giving them a percentage of the office, they want to keep the overhead low. Using the labs that give us discounts makes them win even more, because their quarterly bonus check will be higher if the lab fees are lower.

If the new associate is new in town, they're not going to know any of the specialists. It's really important to get them connected with the specialists so that they're comfortable and can talk intelligently to patients about who they're referring to. We recommend sending a letter to the specialists in the area introducing the new associate, so that specialist can reach out to them personally and ideally set a time to take them out to lunch to get to know them. We all know this is critical to having a proper hand-off and to developing trust in the specialist we are recommending.

Finally, it's important to talk about what expectations you have, as a group, from the associate. We are a very goal-driven organization, and we create a daily goal with our offices, which is tied to a monthly and quarterly bonus. Our Production Division sits down with the associate and creates their daily goal prior to their start. It's critical to communicate this to make sure it's an appropriate goal, but also so the associate understands there's a monthly bonus and that they are a part of that.

It's important to talk about case acceptance and the process we use to try to increase case acceptance. The doctor is going to be involved in the process between the hygienist and the patient care coordinator to develop trust and rapport, and to encourage patients towards accepting treatment. The new associate needs to see their role and needs to be enrolled in that communication process. At first, you can expect new associates to have a lower case acceptance rate than the senior dentist. So the more time you can put into this to offset that difference, the faster the practice will grow and hit bonus.

In the first three months with an associate, our Quality Assurance Division closely monitors online reviews related to the associate. Obviously, all negative reviews should be responded to immediately, but it's important to communicate all reviews to the associate so that they know your eyes are on the reviews and that you're monitoring what patients are saying about them. This will give them just a little added accountability to make sure they're providing a world-class experience right off the bat.

Furthermore, you need to communicate that you're going to be doing clinical audits on the associate, and that you expect world-class dentistry. The senior dentist is going to be assigned to audit the dentist on a regular basis for the first year. They're going to be auditing the quality of dentistry from a dentist's perspective. It's important that you communicate that this is in the spirit of being able to help guide them to become better clinical dentists.

Finally, our Quality Assurance Division meets with the Team Leader every week of the first three months to get feedback on the associate. Again, communicate this to everyone, and emphasize that it's in the spirit of ensuring a world-class environment.

APPENDIX

DIAGRAMS 1 - 16

Bookkeeping Process

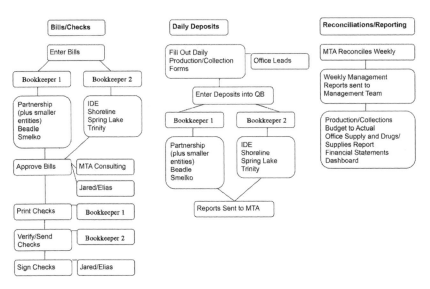

Diagram 1a: Centralized Bookkeeping Work Tree

Payroll Process

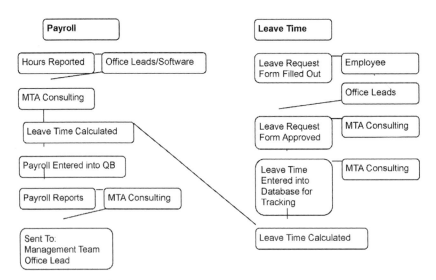

Diagram 1b: Centralized Payroll Work Tree

Appendix

Human Resources Process

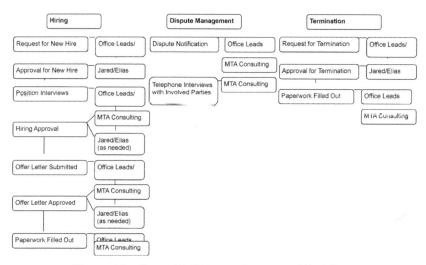

Diagram 1c: Centralized Human Resources Work Tree

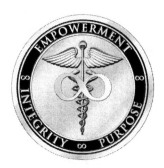

Diagram 2: IDP Corporate Coin

Thu, Mar 31, 3:41 PM

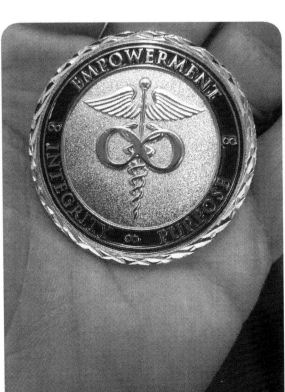

Had to have a tough, unpleasant conversation today, but I brought this, and it gave me the confidence I needed to get it done. Thanks guys. I'm grateful for where we've been, and hopeful for where we're going.

Diagram 3: Associate Message Utilizing Coin

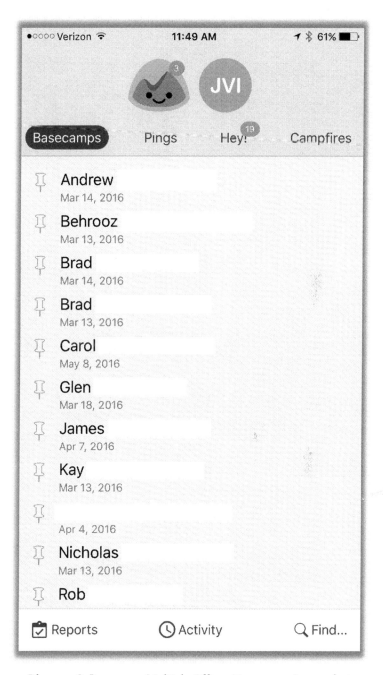

Diagram 4: Basecamp Multiple Offices Homepage Screenshot

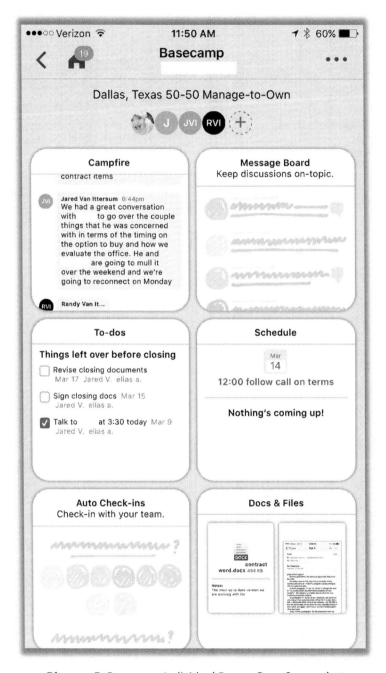

Diagram 5: Basecamp Individual Doctor Page Screenshot

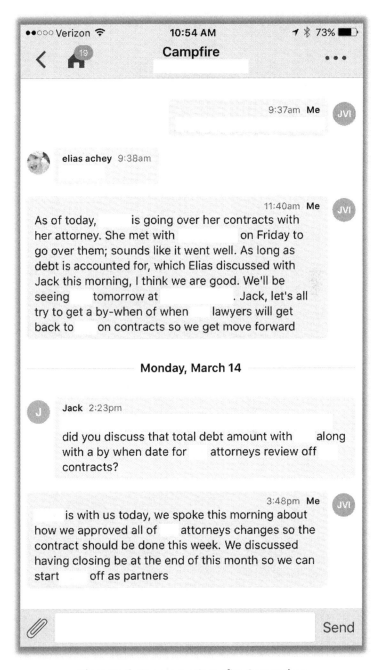

Diagram 6: Basecamp Campfire Screenshot

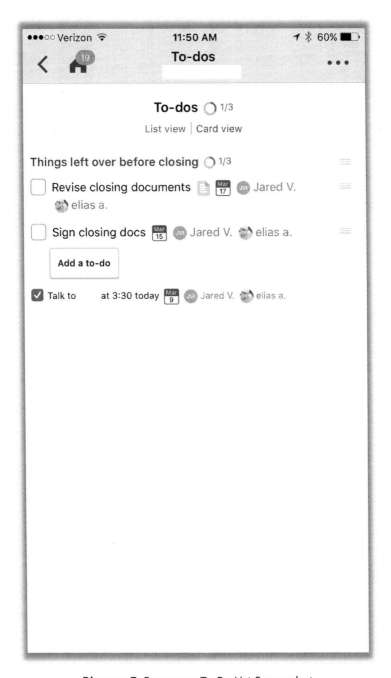

Diagram 7: Basecamp To Do List Screenshot

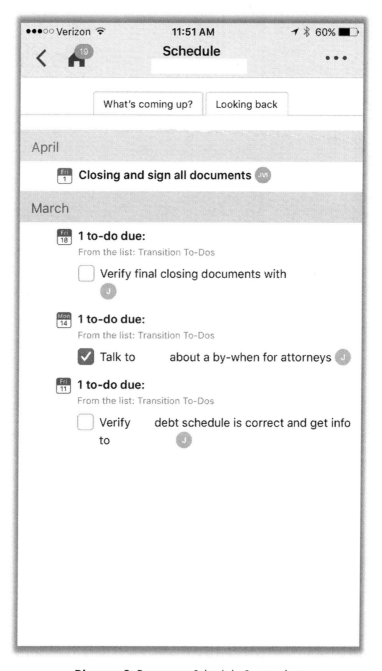

Diagram 8: Basecamp Schedule Screenshot

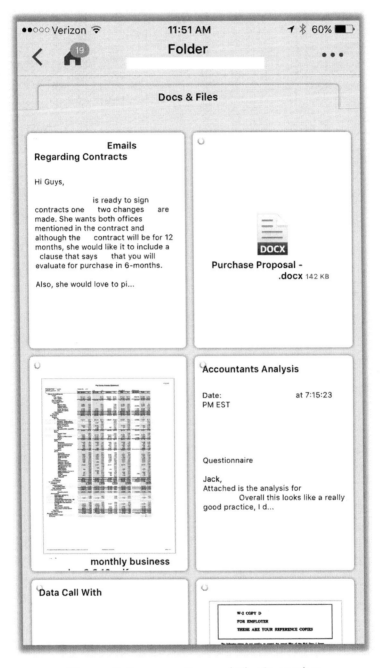

Diagram 9: Basecamp Docs and Files Screenshot

answerconnect ≡

If you like to get in contact with an AnswerConnect representative please consider giving us a call, chat or email.

Sales

For question regarding services and offerings or custom quotes please contact us and one of our friendly sales reps will happy to assist you.

sales@answerconnect.com

866.332.3935

Client Services

If you are an existing customer and need assistance with your account setup, maintenance, billing or online access please contact our client services department.

clientservices@answerconnect.com

800.531.5828

Diagram 10: AnswerConnect Contact Page Screenshot

data collection Sun. July 29th 2012

- Collections:780000 on track for 1M This year.

- Active Patients: 2800

- Ins. Fee for service ppo:fee for service

- % of collections from hygiene: 29.3%

- # of hygienist: 2 full

- # Hygiene days: 8

- Dental assistant:2 full

- Associates: no dr.   works 4 days a week

- # New patients / month:

- type of marketing used now:outside none

- # of opertories: 5

- Room for additional opps. (unused): 2 plumbed & wired

- Monitors in opps: yes 1

- Software in use:dentrics

- Digital x-rays:no

- Digital pan:no

Diagram 11a: Doctor Summary Email from Acquisition Team -Part A

- Inter oral cameras:yes

- Cerec:no

- E4D:no

- Sq. ft. of bldg. 3300

- Own or lease: own

- If own would you lease or sell: both

- Demographics of your patients: all walks of life

- Years in present area and population:2 (17) 10,000 ppl greater metro area 300,000 ppl

- Largest metropolitan near you: 290,000 ppl, 10 mi. away

- Years in practice: 36

- How many yrs have passed since you were born:66

- **Misc. notes** bought an existing practice in 95, in 2004 brought in an associate who wanted to buy the practice. The new associate got into some difficulties and asked to hold off on the sale for a time. In 2007 the associate bought practice and stayed on.

Diagram 11b: Doctor Summary Email from Acquisition Team -Part B

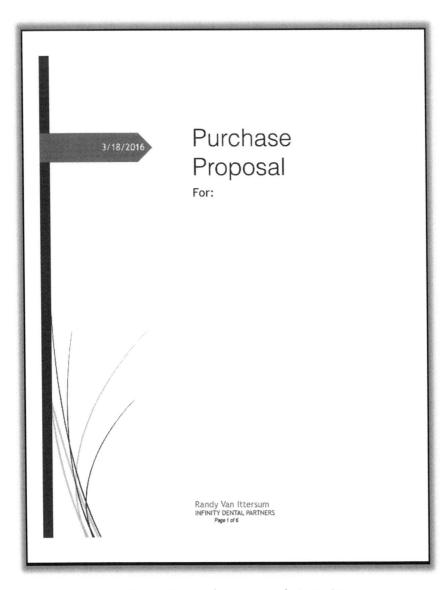

Diagram 12: Practice Purchase Proposal - Front Cover

Dear Dr. ,

I am contacting you on behalf of my son, Dr. Jared Van Ittersum and his partner Dr. Elias Achey.

They asked me to find ten dentists in your state that would be interested in affiliating with a large group practice that is the anti-cola of corporate dentistry, recognizes and supports the unique DNA of each dental office, and believes that nothing will ever replace quality, personalized dental care.

They are looking for three types (groups) of dentists.

1. A dentist who is interested in owning MULTIPLE dental practices and would entertain partnering with an organization that has created the blueprint for developing and managing a large group practice.

2. A dentist who is TIRED and FRUSTRATED with managing his/her practice, has hit a ceiling on his/her income and would like a partner who has skin in the game, and wants to double the size of your practice in the next 2-3 years.

3. A dentist who is thinking about TRANSITIONING out of his/her practice in the next 10 years, and wants a built in buyer when he/she is ready to slow down or retire.

If any of these opportunities are of interest to you, and you would like to have a further conversation, please email me at randy@infinitydentalpartners.com or call Jack Stevens or myself at 616-877-9097.

Sincerely,

Randy Van Ittersum

On behalf of Jared M. Van Ittersum, D.D.S. and Elias Achey, D.M.D.

Confidential

Diagram 13: Picture of our Direct Mailer Letter

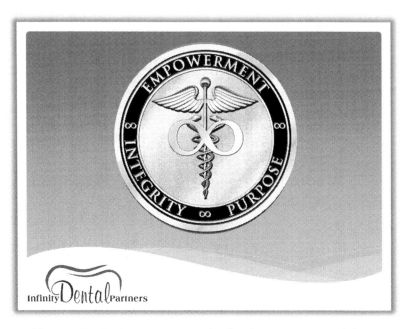

Diagram 14: IDP Doctor Presentation for Group Practice – Slide 01

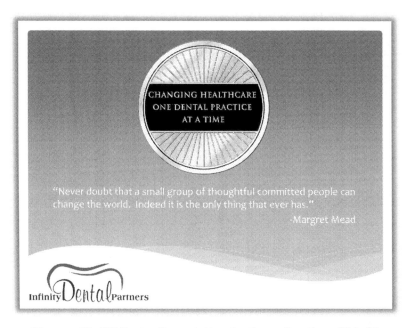

Diagram 14: IDP Doctor Presentation for Group Practice – Slide 02

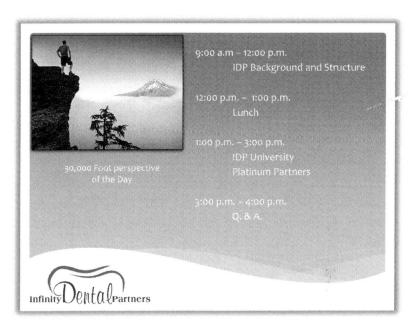

Diagram 14: IDP Doctor Presentation for Group Practice – Slide 03

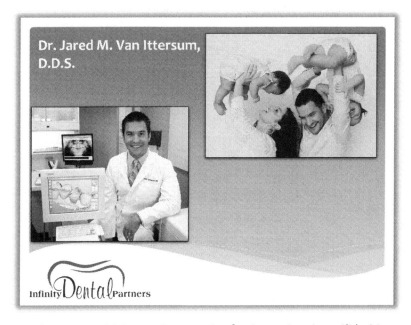

Diagram 14: IDP Doctor Presentation for Group Practice – Slide 04

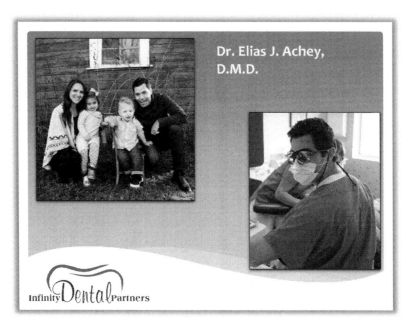

Diagram 14: IDP Doctor Presentation for Group Practice – Slide 05

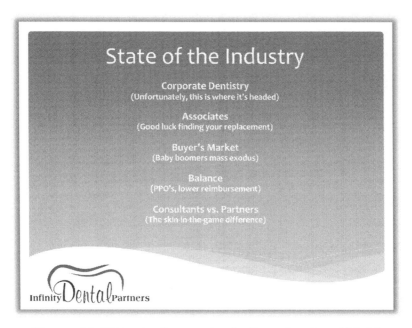

Diagram 14: IDP Doctor Presentation for Group Practice – Slide 06

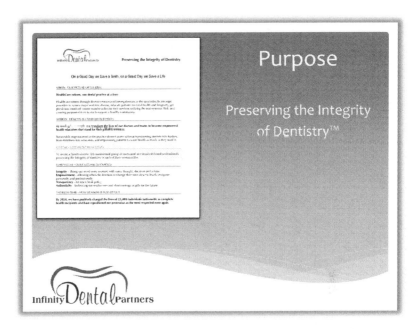

Diagram 14: IDP Doctor Presentation for Group Practice – Slide 07

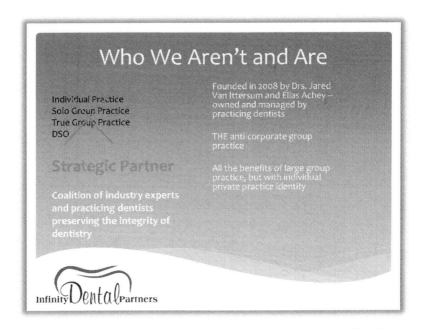

Diagram 14: IDP Doctor Presentation for Group Practice – Slide 08

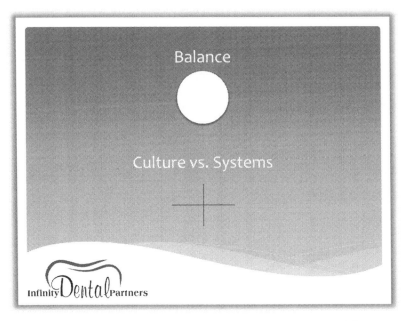

Diagram 14: IDP Doctor Presentation for Group Practice – Slide 09

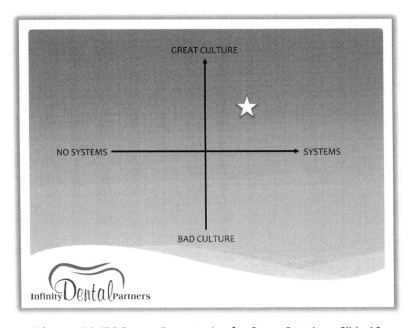

Diagram 14: IDP Doctor Presentation for Group Practice – Slide 10

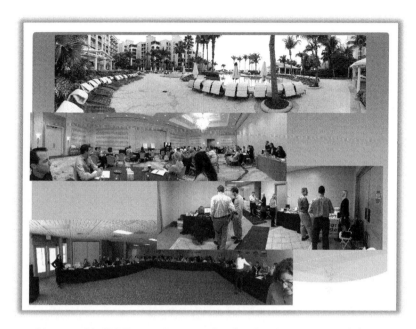

Diagram 14: IDP Doctor Presentation for Group Practice – Slide 11

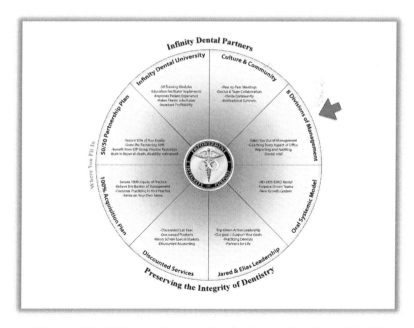

Diagram 14: IDP Doctor Presentation for Group Practice – Slide 12

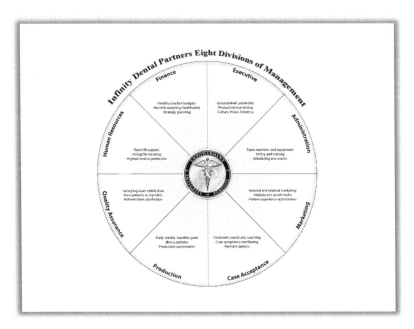

Diagram 14: IDP Doctor Presentation for Group Practice – Slide 13

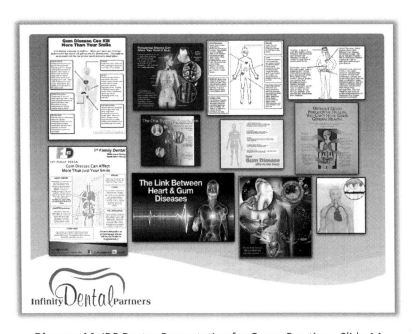

Diagram 14: IDP Doctor Presentation for Group Practice – Slide 14

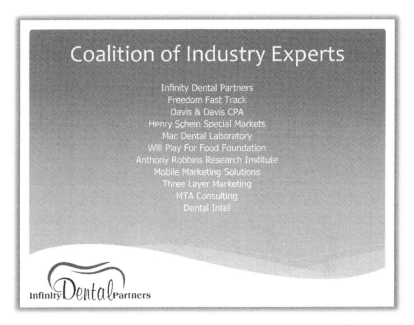

Diagram 14: IDP Doctor Presentation for Group Practice – Slide 15

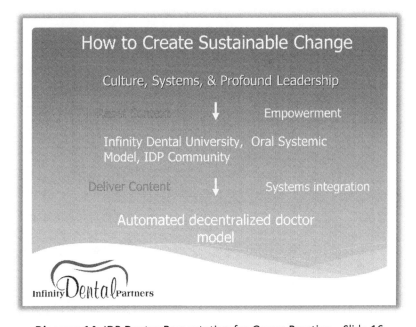

Diagram 14: IDP Doctor Presentation for Group Practice – Slide 16

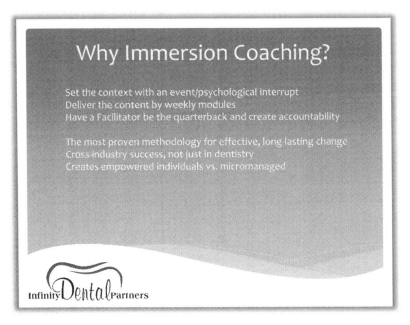

Diagram 14: IDP Doctor Presentation for Group Practice – Slide 17

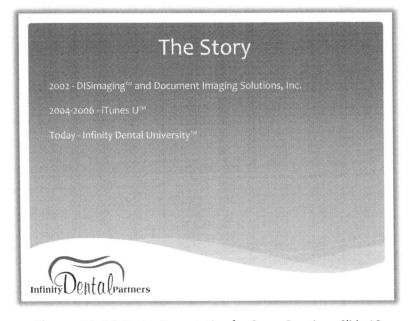

Diagram 14: IDP Doctor Presentation for Group Practice – Slide 18

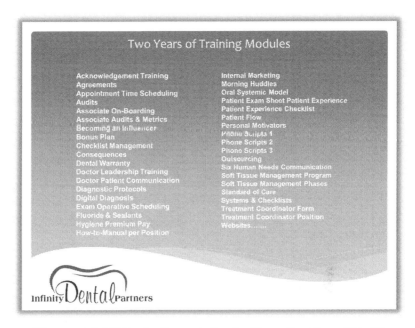

Diagram 14: IDP Doctor Presentation for Group Practice – Slide 19

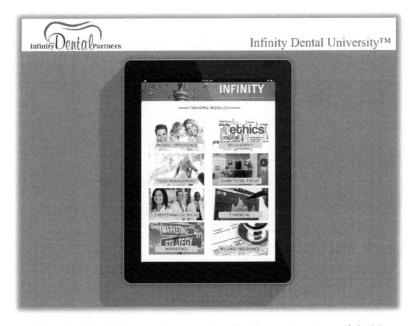

Diagram 14: IDP Doctor Presentation for Group Practice – Slide 20

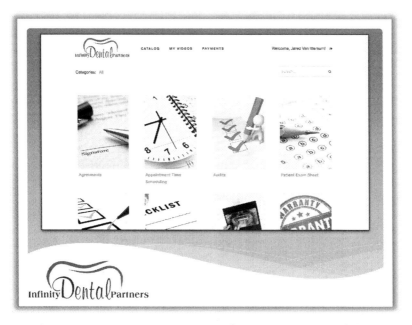

Diagram 14: IDP Doctor Presentation for Group Practice – Slide 21

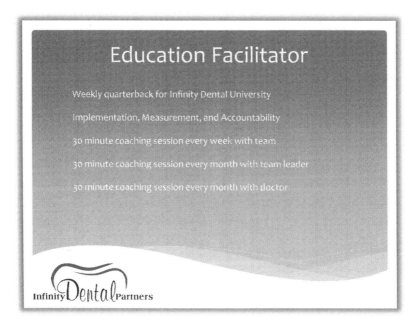

Diagram 14: IDP Doctor Presentation for Group Practice – Slide 22

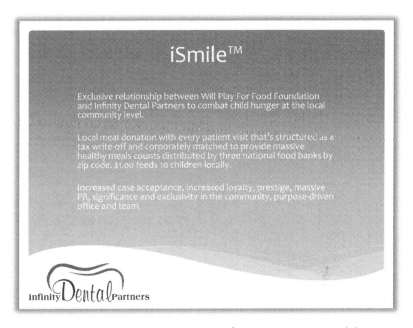

Diagram 14: IDP Doctor Presentation for Group Practice – Slide 23

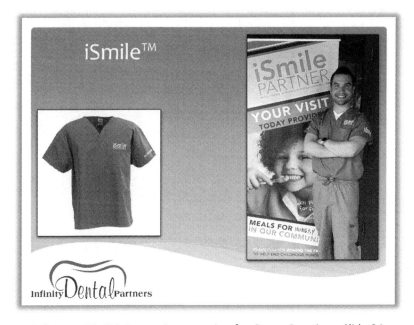

D iagram 14: IDP Doctor Presentation for Group Practice – Slide 24

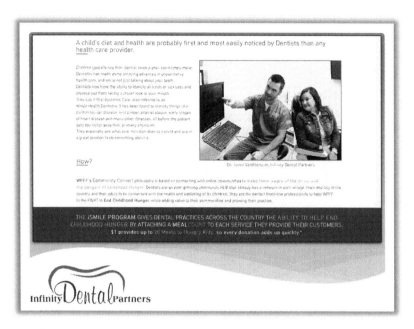

Diagram 14: IDP Doctor Presentation for Group Practice – Slide 25

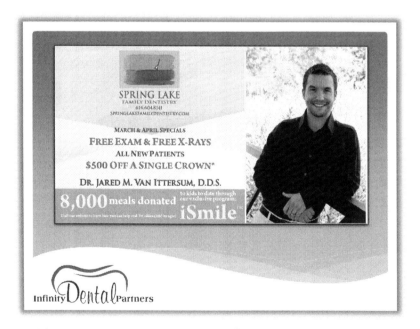

Diagram 14: IDP Doctor Presentation for Group Practice – Slide 26

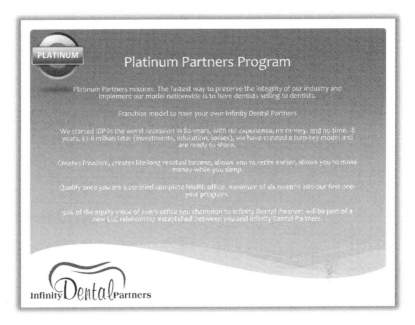

Diagram 14: IDP Doctor Presentation for Group Practice – Slide 27

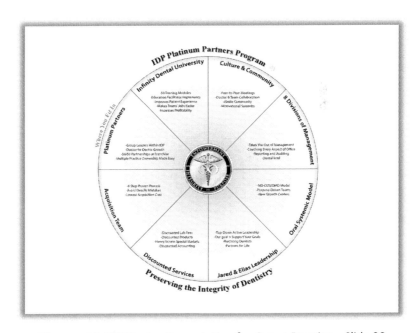

Diagram 14: IDP Doctor Presentation for Group Practice – Slide 28

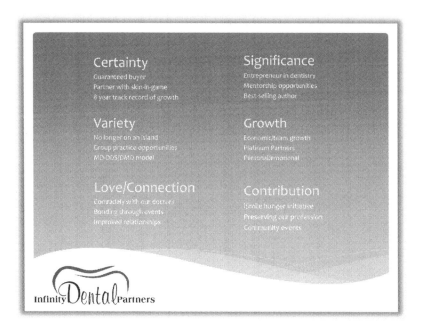

Diagram 14: IDP Doctor Presentation for Group Practice – Slide 29

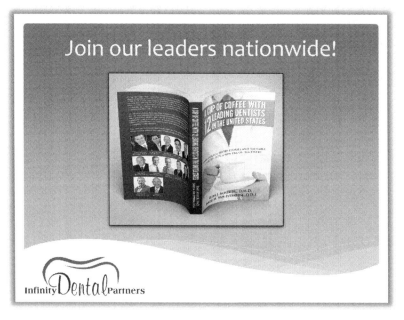

Diagram 14: IDP Doctor Presentation for Group Practice – Slide 30

Mission Vision Core Values Statement Exercise

1. **Mission - The "Why" or "Reason" the office exists**
   a. Why are you in business? Wellness, take care of needs, change lives, best care in those of need, devotion to dentistry, educated, provide a need in healthcare, exceptional dental access, healthcare and oral care, to provide dental needs, for the love of people.
   b. How would you like your patients to view you? Honest, compassionate, trustworthy, nurturing, authentic, genuine, quality time, friendly, state of-art, skillful, courteous, professional, friendly.
   c. What level of service do you wish to provide? Quality, compassionate, highest level, superior, exceptional, optimal, maximum wellness, dependable, excellent service.
   d. Outside your core business, what else would you like your practice to be known for? caring for homeless, caring for schools, outreach, missionary, community, confidential connection, stuartship, relaxation, peacefulness, accountability, quality service, honest compassionate.
   e. How are you different from your competitors? Laid back, fun atmosphere, go out of way for patients, personal touch, highly personalized, service before self, integrity first, meaningful relationships, providing life services, oral-systemic, 15 years of service in community, multi speciality practice, your dental home, more service oriented, family oriented, well-known dentistry, referrals, down to earth, family atmosphere, above and beyond.

   Our Mission: We change lives with compassion, integrity and a superior personal touch in a state-of-the-art multi specialty practice.

2. **Vision - "Where" your office is going.**
   a. What will the practice look like in five to ten years? Mastered, Polished, united as a team, full time, fully functional surgical suite, group of expanded offices, benefits and bonus, exponential growth, fulfilling the communities needs, fully optimized space, nationally recognized brand, state-of-the-art, highly productive
   b. How will the community perceive us in five to ten years? The best, all inclusive care, #1 cosmetic, ER care, Popular, Pioneering, constant, offering state of the art services.
   c. What will be our market position in five to ten years? Education, #1 affordable private practice, top 1% in   stability, patient approved
   d. How will we remain true to our Mission Statement as we grow? Loyalty to patients, steadfast, daily affirmation, through positive experiences, accountability, self growth.

   Our Vision: Fulfilling the communities needs as a nationally recognized patient approved private practice group through positive experiences.

3. **Core Values**
   a. What are your three core values as a team? integrity, authenticity, impeccable, polished, purpose, service before self, excellence, admirable

   Our core values: Excellence, integrity, authenticity

102 S. Buchanan, Spring Lake, MI 49456   www.infinitydentalpartners.com

Diagram 15: Mission Vision Purpose Value Statement Exercise Example

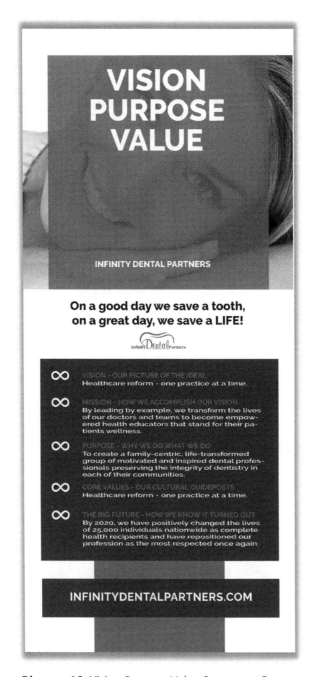

Diagram 16: Vision Purpose Value Statement Banner

32512833R00117

Made in the USA
Middletown, DE
07 June 2016